肺部双重供血 CT 灌注原理及临床应用

THE PRINCIPLE AND CLINICAL APPLICATION OF DUAL – INPUT CT PERFUSION IN LUNG

主 编 袁小东 敖国昆

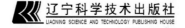

辽宁科学技术出版社
LIAONING SCIENCE AND TECHNOLOGY PUBLISHING HOUSE

内容简介

本书作者长期从事肺部疾病影像学诊断及 CT 灌注技术研究，于 2011 年开发了肺部双重供血 CT 灌注技术，该技术通过宽体探测器 CT 肺部动态容积扫描获得肺循环和体循环血流动力学参数，对肺肿瘤的良恶性鉴别及抗肿瘤血管生成药物的疗效监测有重要价值。

本书详细阐述了肺部双重供血 CT 灌注技术的原理并展示了大量的临床病例，全面、新颖，图文并茂，可供医疗机构影像科、呼吸科、胸外科医师及大学科研机构研究人员使用。

图书在版编目（CIP）数据

肺部双重供血 CT 灌注原理及临床应用/袁小东，敖国昆主编. —沈阳：辽宁科学技术出版社，2018.7

ISBN 978 - 7 - 5381 - 9999 - 4

Ⅰ. ①肺… Ⅱ. ①袁… ②敖… Ⅲ. ①肺部双重供血 CT Ⅳ. ①R791.5

中国版本图书馆 CIP 数据核字（2016）第 24581 号

出版发行：辽宁科学技术出版社
　　　　　（地址：沈阳市和平区十一纬路 29 号 邮编：110003）
联系电话：010-57262361/024-23284376
E - mail：fushimedbook@163.com
印 刷 者：三河市双峰印刷装订有限公司
经 销 者：各地新华书店

幅面尺寸：185mm×260mm
字　　数：250 千字　　　　　　　　　　印　张：9
出版时间：2018 年 8 月第 1 版　　　　　印刷时间：2018 年 8 月第 1 次印刷

责任编辑：李俊卿　　　　　　　　　　　责任校对：梁晓洁
封面设计：永诚天地　　　　　　　　　　封面制作：永诚天地
版式设计：天地鹏博　　　　　　　　　　责任印制：丁 艾

如有质量问题，请速与印务部联系 联系电话：010-57262361

定　　价：120.00 元

《肺部双重供血 CT 灌注原理及临床应用》
编 委 会

主编简介

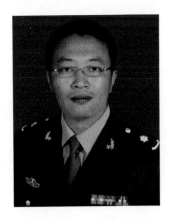

　　袁小东，男，1976 年出生，江苏东台人，第二军医大学医学博士，解放军 309 医院放射科副主任医师，硕士生导师。长期从事 CT 灌注研究，于 2011 年开发肺部双重供血 CT 灌注技术（Dual－input CT perfusion，DI－CTP），相关 CT 灌注研究发表在影像医学顶级期刊 Radiology 和 European Radiology 杂志上，被国内外广泛引用。CT 灌注能够测量肺及肺部病灶的体循环和肺循环的血流量，揭示病变的血流动力学特征，对包括肺癌在内的各种肺部疾病的诊断及疗效评估有较大帮助。作者目前主持国家自然科学基金面上项目、北京市科委"首都临床特色应用"课题、军队干部保健专项等课题。兼任中国研究型医院学会放射专业青年委员会副主任委员、白求恩医学专家青年科学家委员会常务委员，享受军队优秀专业技术人才岗位津贴。

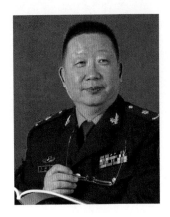

　　敖国昆，主任医师，医学硕士，硕士生导师，解放军 309 医院放射科主任。中国研究型医院学会放射学专业委员会副主任委员兼秘书长，中国研究型医院学会介入专业委员会副主任委员，防痨协会临床专业委员会影像组副组长，全军放射诊断设备质量安全控制委员会副主任委员，全军放射专业委员会委员，全军介入专业委员会常委。

前 言 PREFACE

　　肺由体循环和肺循环供血，生理状态下肺循环占绝对优势，病理状态下体循环有较强可塑性，肺癌主要由体循环供血，但所占比例不甚明确，以往缺乏有效手段判断其血供来源及量化体、肺循环的比例，因此能定量评估肺癌体、肺循环的影像手段具有重要临床应用价值；由于肺部良、恶性病灶的形态学征象重叠较多，鉴别诊断一直是影像医学的难点之一，双重供血 CT 灌注技术能够提供形态学以外的血流动力学信息，对肺部病灶的定性诊断会有所帮助。本书作者长期从事肺部疾病影像学诊断及 CT 灌注技术研究，于 2011 年开发了肺部双重供血 CT 灌注技术，该技术通过宽体探测器 CT 肺部动态容积扫描获得肺循环和体循环血流动力学参数，对肺肿瘤的良恶性鉴别及抗肿瘤血管生成药物的疗效监测有重要价值。

　　本书详细阐述了肺部双重供血 CT 灌注技术的原理并展示了大量的临床病例，知识新颖，图文并茂，可供医疗机构影像科、呼吸科、胸外科医师及大学科研机构研究人员使用。

袁小东

2018 年 5 月

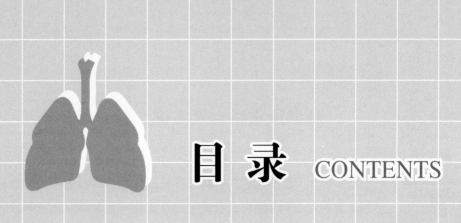

目 录 CONTENTS

第三章

肺部双重供血 CT 灌注技术临床研究

第四章

肺双重供血 CT 灌注技术临床病例展示

第一章

对比剂首过 CT 灌注成像技术概述

20 世纪 90 年代末到 2000 年，电子束 CT 使用定量分析的动态首过增强灌注 CT 在动物和正常人及肺栓塞患者的研究被报道。之后，多排螺旋 CT（multidetector row CT，MDCT）的临床应用，使得动态首过增强灌注 CT 在 MDCT 上得以实施[1,2]。MDCT 灌注成像技术能显示，组织的灌注状态且能进一步进行定量分析，使得组织内部血流动力学研究有了新的手段，诸多研究显示，利用 MDCT 首过动态增强灌注的定量方法对肺部肿瘤或孤立性结节进行定性或对肺癌患者接受保守治疗的疗效评价非常有潜力[3-7]。

MDCT 的面世使得 CT 扫描的空间分辨力及时间分辨力大大提高，能够及时捕获到注射对比剂后数十秒内靶器官及其供血动脉的增强信息，绘制出相应的时间密度曲线（time density curve，TDC）。依据质量守恒定理、中央容积定理及对比剂稀释原理可进一步计算出组织的血流灌注值（blood flow，BF）、组织血容量（blood volume，BV）、对比剂平均通过时间（mean transit time，MTT）。临床常用动态扫描技术：团注适量对比剂后延迟数秒或十数秒后启动扫描，固定于某一层面或某几个层面进行快速连续扫描。由灌注软件给出彩色灌注图，也可手工描绘出兴趣区（region of interest，ROI），计算相应的血流灌注参数[8]。

计算灌注值常用的数学模型有：最大斜率法（maximal slop method）、对比剂平衡原理、去卷积算法（deconvolution）。其中以 Miles 等[9]提出的最大斜率法和去卷积算法最为常用[10,11]。最大斜率法事先假设在主动脉增强达峰值时静脉内尚未有对比剂流出，理论上要求更高的对比剂注射流率，而去卷积算法对对比剂注射流率的要求不高，没有对灌注模型做过多假设，理论上在低速率注射条件下可以实现血流灌注的准确测量，实践也证明所得结果与实际生理过程更为接近。

第一节　去卷积算法在 CT 灌注中的应用

大多数组织灌注测量模型建立在以下相似的理论模型及假设的基础上：所检测脏器或组织的血流供应有一个或数个进口，一个出口，进口的流入量（速率）等于出口的流出量（速率）；所用造影剂为血池型造影剂，不会穿过毛细血管壁弥散到组织间隙中去；只要观察时间足够长，进入组织的造影剂分子终会从静脉流出（认为组织不会摄取造影剂分子）；单位体积组织中造影剂的含量和组织的 CT 增加值成正比，经测算每毫克碘可使一毫升组织的 CT 值升高约 25 Hu[12]。根据 Ficker 原理，某一时刻 t 流入组织的造影剂总量减去流出组织的造影剂总量等于组织内的造影剂剩余量 Q（质量守恒定理），用公式表示为：

$$F \cdot \left[\int_0^t a(t)\,dt - \int_0^t v(t)\,dt \right] = Q \tag{1}$$

Miles 等提出的最大斜率法即在以上基础上进一步假设注射造影剂后短时间内未有造影剂流出组织，这时公式（1）变为：

$$F \cdot \int_0^t a(t)\,dt = Q(t)$$

进一步可得：

$$F = Q(t) \cdot a(t)^{-1}$$

即组织血流量近似等于组织强化初始段的最大斜率除以主动脉的强化峰值。这就要求最大斜率的测量点必须在最小通过时间前，如脑组织的最小通过时间为 3～5s，这在实际临床应用中往往要求注射速度达到 10 ml/s 以上，增加了患者的检查风险。

考虑到去卷积算法没有对灌注模型做过多假设，理论上在低速率注射条件下可以实现血流灌注的准确测量。为了验证这一方法假设的准确性，本书作者在 2004 年通过采集 30 例健康成人的肾脏皮质 MDCT 灌注扫描数据，采用去卷积算法计算灌注参数，由所得参数进一步推算肾静脉增强 TDC，并与实际测得肾静脉 TDC 进行比较，计算决定系数 R^2，评价两者的吻合程度。结果显示，理论计算所得肾静脉 TDC 与实测 TDC 符合程度较高（R^2 均数的95% CI 0.85～0.91），从而说明在 CT 组织灌注测量中去卷积算法是一种较准确的计算方法[13]。下面将这一研究内容进行详细介绍。

1 资料与方法

1.1 研究对象 30 例健康成人，男 18 名，女 12 名，年龄 30～40 岁，行左肾静脉水平的 CT 动态灌注扫描（考虑左肾静脉走行较水平，易于在横断面内显示）。

1.2 成像方法 CT 机型为 Siemens Somatom plus 4，对比剂采用优维显，每例40 ml，自肘静脉注入，速率为 4 ml/s。扫描序列为 Body perfusion，准直器宽度为 5 mm，120 kV，300 mA，层厚为 5 mm，4 层，定位在左肾静脉水平，扫描周期为 1 s，每例扫 40 层，延迟 6 s，屏气扫描，挑选肾静脉最宽层面进行灌注测量。分别在腹主动脉（代替肾动脉）、左肾静脉及左肾皮质内画感兴趣区。画感兴趣区时注意与脏器边缘保持适当距离，以减少部分容积效应的影响，在此前提下争取尽可能大的面积以提高信噪比。

1.3 统计分析 利用工作站 Dynamic Evaluation 软件得出相应的时间密度曲线（time - density - curve，TDC）并导出数据，由 Visual Basic 语言编写的应用程序完成去卷积运算（数学方法参照 Cuenod 等[14]），得出血流量（BF）、平均通过时间（mean transit time，MTT）、血容量（blood volume，BV）及脉冲剩余函数 R（t）（impulse residue function），由 R（t）计算出 h（t），并与腹主动脉 TDC 卷积得出理论上的肾静脉 TDC，然后与实际测得的肾静脉 TDC 比较，以理论计算值作为实测值的拟合曲线，计算决定系数 R^2，评价两者的吻合程度，$R^2 \geq 0.85$ 者认为吻合较好。统计工作在 MS Excel 2000 中完成。

2　结果

左肾血流量为（4.2±0.4）ml/（min·ml），血容量为 0.77±0.06，平均通过时间平均值为（12.49±1.3）s，肾静脉拟合的决定系数为 0.88±0.08（表 1）。决定系数 R^2 均数的 95% 的可信区间为 0.85~0.91。

表 1　30 例左肾皮质 CT 灌注的统计结果

指标	均数	标准差	95% 可信区间	
			下限	上限
BF	4.20	0.40	4.04	4.36
MTT	12.49	1.30	11.98	13.00
BV	0.77	0.06	0.75	0.79
R2	0.88	0.08	0.85	0.91

单位：BF：ml/（min ml）；MTT、BV：ml/g

3　去卷积算法准确性验证分析

本研究采用经左肾静脉平面的 CT 灌注扫描。肾皮质的血流量占整个肾血流量的 95% 以上，本研究没有考虑肾髓质灌注对肾静脉内对比剂浓度的影响。进入肾动脉的血流有两个去向，大部分回流入肾静脉，少部分经肾血管球滤出至肾球囊腔，经近端肾小管、远端肾小管、集合管，最终至肾盏、肾盂形成尿液。肾血管球、肾球囊及近端肾小管几乎全部位于肾皮质内，在 CT 灌注扫描的时段内（本研究为 0~40 s），认为尚没有造影剂经肾小管或集合管到达肾髓质内（分析 30 例 body perfusion 的原始图像也未发现肾髓质的明显强化），这是本实验的数学模型得以成立的前提。

Silverman 和 Burgen 等[15]在 20 世纪 60 年代最早把卷积原理引入活体血管内血药浓度研究中。造影剂或药物由动脉输入，其浓度函数为 a（t），组织内的剩余造影剂浓度函数为 Q（t），静脉端的输出浓度函数为 v（t），此输入—输出系统可以看成一个线性系统（linear system）[16]，对任何一个脉冲式的输入系统有一个固定的反应函数 h（t）与之相对应（图 1，2）。如某个瞬时输入量为 q，系统对此做出反应产生输出函数为 q·h（t）。h（t）是由系统的内部属性决定的，反映了所研究系统的属性，从统计学的角度可以理解为：示踪造影剂分子在 0 时刻从动脉端以脉冲式注入后随机分散在"迷宫"一样的组织微血管内，经过一段时间（最小通过时间），第一个造影剂分子跑出组织进入静脉端，随后静脉端造影剂浓度越来越高，并达到一个峰值，接着逐渐衰减至 0（图 5）。

叠加原理（superposition principle）是线性系统的重要特征。可以用如下两种情况加以阐述：①某一瞬时动脉端的输入量为 2q，其静脉端的输出函数等于输入量为 q 时的两次代数叠加（图 1，2）。②三次量子式输入时间间隔为 dt，每次剂量为 q，其静脉端的输出函数为单次输入剂量为 q 时的输出函数加上两个依次后推 dt 时间间隔所得函数的代数和（图 3，4），此处把最小通过时间假设为 0。循此推理，当输入函数 a（t）为任意连续函数时输出函数记为：

$$v(t) = a(t) \cdot h(t) = \int_0^t a(\tau) \cdot h(t-\tau) \cdot d\tau \qquad (2)$$

其中 * 号为卷积算子，$\tau \in [0, t]$。如果已知 a（t）和 v（t）则 h（t）可以用卷积算法的逆运算（去卷积）来表示：

$$h（t）= v（t）// a（t） \qquad (3)$$

其中"//"是去卷积运算符。卷积的计算表达式是一个较复杂的积分形式，在计算时常进行 Laplace 转换[17]。

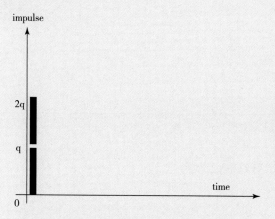

图 1　输入函数为脉冲式，0 时刻大小为 q 或 2q

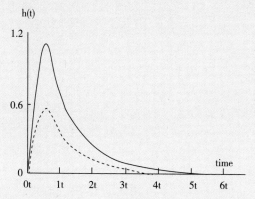

图 2　对应图（1），输出函数为 qh（t）或 2qh（t）

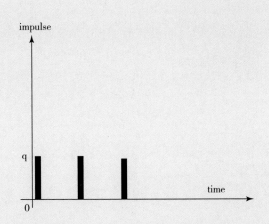

图 3　输入函数为脉冲式，在三个不同时刻大小都为 **q**，时间间隔为 **dt**

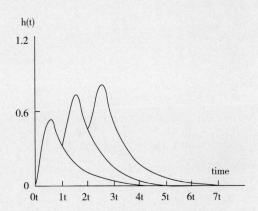

图 4　对应图（3），输出函数为三次脉冲式输入的代数和

　　研究在体组织的血流灌注也就是寻找反映组织血流动力学属性的反应函数 h（t）的过程（图 5）。在实际应用中容易在某一断层内找到所研究组织的供血动脉，但往往很难找到它的引流静脉，即便有也常常不能用来计算输出函数，因为静脉血内的造影剂常常来自多个组织或脏器。这种情况就变成了已知输入函数 a（t），即动脉 TDC 和组织的 CT 增强函数 CTp，即组织感兴趣区 TDC，求 h（t）。因 h（t）代表了脉冲式输入后 t 时刻出口处造影剂的浓度，其积分形式 H（t）代表了 t 时刻已由出口流出的造影剂的量，1−H（t）就代表了 t 时刻滞留在组织中的造影剂的量，用脉冲剩余函数 R（t）（impulse residue function）表示[16]，它同样反映了组织的血流动力学属性。经与上文相似的推理可得如下公式：

$$CT_P = F \cdot a（t）\cdot R（t）= a（t）\cdot F \cdot R（t） \tag{4}$$

$$F \cdot R（t）= CT_p // a（t） \tag{5}$$

CT_p 为组织的 CT 增强函数，单位为 Hu，F 为组织的血流量（blood flow），理论上 R（t）的曲线形态（图6）有一个平台期，高度为1，接着是一个衰减期，最终无限接近于 X 轴，时段 t＋dt 内流出组织的造影剂为阴影部分所代表，其通过时间近似为 t，整个曲线可以分割成无限多个 d t，因此所有造影剂分子的平均通过时间为整个曲线下的面积，即：

$$MTT = \int_0^\infty R(t)\,dt \tag{6}$$

如 F · R（t）已求出，其平台期的高度值（F）即为 BF，依据中央容积定理，组织血容量可以由下式求出：

$$BV = BF \cdot MTT \tag{7}$$

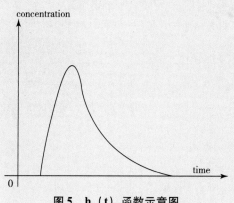

图5　h（t）函数示意图

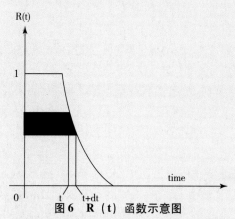

图6　R（t）函数示意图

时段 t＋dt 内流出组织的造影剂为阴影部分所代表

去卷积求解方法：去卷积是卷积的逆运算，类似于乘法和除法的关系，因为已知的组织增强 TDC 和动脉增强 TDC 都是由数据点描绘成的，并不知道其明确的函数表达式，所以不可能用数学方法直接进行去卷积运算，用的较多的方法是先估计一个函数表达式与动脉增强 TDC 进行卷积，看结果是否与组织增强 TDC 相符，找出一个最理想的函数表达式，使卷积结果与组织增强 TDC 符合程度最高，那么这个函数表达式最接近于 F·R（t），可以用它代替 F·R（t）得出组织灌注参数。Cuenod 等[13]用 Weibull 函数代替 F·R（t），因为 Weibull 函数的曲线形态介于指数函数和幂函数之间，最有可能与理论上的 R（t）函数的曲线形态相一致，表达式为：

$$F \cdot R(t) = f \cdot \exp[-(t/b)^c] \tag{8}$$

CT 动态扫描的采样周期设为 T，由公式（4）可以给出组织增强函数的近似计算公式：

$$CT_P = a(nT) \cdot FR(nT) = T \sum_{k=0}^{n-1} a(nT - KT) \cdot FR(KT)$$

$$= T \sum_{k=0}^{n-1} a(nT - KT) \cdot f \cdot \exp[-(KT/b)^c] \tag{9}$$

公式（9）中 f，b，c 为三个未知参数，由电脑程序求解出最合理的数值使得由公式（9）所得曲线与组织感兴趣区 TDC 各数据点之间的残差平方和最小（最小二乘法法则）。理论肾静脉 TDC 的推算及拟合优度评价首先由 R（t）计算出 h（t）：

$$h(t) = -R(t)' \tag{10}$$

理论肾静脉增强 TDC 为腹主动脉 TDC 和 h（t）的卷积（图7），用 v_T（t）表示：

$$v_T(t) = a(t) \cdot h(t) \tag{11}$$

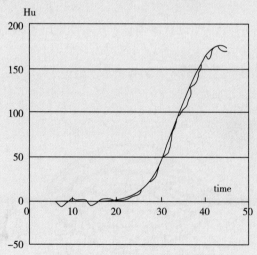

图7　细线为肾静脉 TDC，粗线为腹主动脉 TDC 和
h（t）的卷积，两者吻合程度较高，$R^2 = 0.9$

用决定系数 R^2 来评价理论肾静脉增强 TDC 与实测肾静脉 TDC 吻合程度，计算公式为：

$$R^2 = 1 - \frac{SS_{残}}{SS_{总}} \tag{12}$$

公式中：$SS_残$为残差平方和，$SS_总$为总的离均差平方和。在曲线拟合中决定系数 R^2 通常被用来评价拟合曲线与已知数据资料的吻合程度，其取值范围在 0 ~ 1 之间，值越大说明吻合程度越高。本次研究中决定系数 R^2 的平均值为 0.88，95% 的可信区间为 0.85 ~ 0.91，如以 0.85 为标准，可以认为左肾静脉的理论 TDC 与实际测得的 TDC 吻合程度较高。在同一坐标中观察实测肾静脉 TDC 及理论计算所得肾静脉 TDC 发现，这 30 例的实测数据总体上有略低于理论数据的倾向（图 7），这可能是因为肾静脉的横断面直径偏小，画感兴趣区时虽然已注意避开血管边缘，仍很难排除其上下层面容积效应的影响，或者轻微的呼吸移动也可引起同样的效果，这些因素最终都会导致 R^2 值的减小。

第二节　最大斜率法及改良最大斜率法在 CT 灌注中的应用

去卷积算法理论的合理性及结果的准确性已被越来越多的研究者认可，但计算的复杂性阻碍了其在临床应用及研究中的推广，虽然已有商业化的软件包面世，但同时也带来了检测费用的大幅度上升。同时去卷积算法利用了 TDC 上所有的数据点，为了得到准确可靠的结果，要求 CT 扫描的时间范围为从主动脉增强起点至主动脉峰值以后的一段时间，这样相应也增加了患者的射线剂量。

大多数组织灌注测量模型建立在以下相似的理论模型及假设的基础上：

（1）所检测脏器或组织的血流供应有一个进口，一个出口（图 1 - 2 - 1），进口的流入量（流率）等于出口的流出量（流率）。

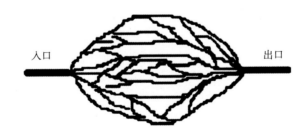

入口　　　　　　　　　　　　　　　　出口

图 1 - 2 - 1　组织灌注示意图

（2）所用对比剂为血池型对比剂，不会穿过毛细血管壁弥散到组织间隙中去。

（3）只要观察时间足够长，进入组织的对比剂分子终会从静脉流出（认为组织不会摄取对比剂分子）。

（4）Ficker 原理，某一时刻 t 流入组织的对比剂总量减去流出组织的对比剂总量等于组织内的对比剂剩余量 CT_p（质量守恒定理）。用公式表示为：

$$F \cdot \left[\int_0^t a(t) - \int_0^t v(t) \right] = CT_P \tag{1}$$

$$F = \frac{CT_P{}'}{a(t) - v(t)} \tag{2}$$

（5）中央容积定理

$$MTT = BV \cdot F^{-1}$$

（6）单位体积组织中对比剂的含量和组织的 CT 增加值成正比，经测算每毫克碘可使 1 ml 组织的 CT 值升高约 25 Hu[12]。

Miles 等提出的最大斜率法就是在以上的基础上进一步假设注射对比剂后短时间内（最小通过时间）没有对比剂流出组织，这时公式（1）变为

$$F = CT_P{}' \cdot a(t)^{-1}$$

即组织血流量近似等于组织强化初始段的最大斜率除以主动脉的强化峰值：

$$F = \frac{最大初始斜率}{主动脉增强峰值} \tag{3}$$

这就要求最大斜率的测量点（理论上与主动脉峰值时间一致），必须在最小通过时间前。如脑组织的最小通过时间为 3 ~ 5 s，在实际临床应用中往往要求注射流率达到 10 ml/s 以上，增加了患者的检查风险。因为理论上的局限性，用最大斜率法计算 BV 和 MTT 需要对灌注模型做进一步的假设，所得结果可靠性较差，实践中较少使用。

改良最大斜率法：在低流率注射条件下，注射同样体积的对比剂后，主动脉的峰值明显后移，主动脉峰值出现时已有对比剂从引流静脉流出，这样最大斜率法的理论假设就不成立，这种情况下组织增强 TDC 的最大斜率点往往比主动脉的强化峰值出现时间要早。由公式（2）及实例观察可以得出这个结论（图 1 - 2 - 2），这时以最大初始斜率除以主动脉强化峰值来计算灌注值就会产生明显的低估。而按公式（4）来计算就较合理，虽然这样不能完全避免对灌注值的低估，因为理论上组织增强 TDC 的最大斜率点在主动脉和引流静脉 C T 值的增速相等的时刻，并不是在引流静脉内刚出现对比剂的时刻。与最大斜率法相似，改良最大斜率法也不太适合于求解 BV 和 MTT。

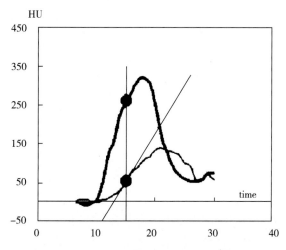

图 1 - 2 - 2　改良最大斜率法手工计算图

$$F = \frac{最大初始斜率}{同时刻主动脉增强值} \tag{4}$$

相比之下，去卷积是卷积的逆运算，是较复杂的积分形式，去卷积算法把组织的微循环看成一个线性系统[17]，对于线性系统，脉冲剩余函数 R（t）（impulse residue function）[14]（图1-2-3）反映了所研究系统（组织）的血流动力学特征，求解的重点在求解 R（t）函数的表达式，通过 R（t）函数可进一步求解出组织灌注参数（BF，BV，MTT），求解过程由 windows 应用程序完成。与最大斜率法不同的是去卷积算法没有预先对灌注模型做过多不合理的假设，其结果的准确性不受对比剂注射流率大小的影响。

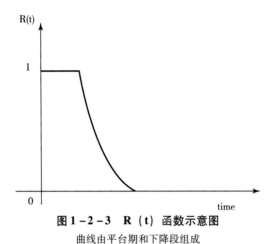

图1-2-3 R（t）函数示意图
曲线由平台期和下降段组成

2004年本书作者[18]为了验证改良最大斜率法在低注射流率时 CT 灌注的准确性，分别以4 ml/s 和2 ml/s 的流率注入对比剂，行灌注扫描，分析了40例健康成人双肾皮质 CT 灌注数据，选择最大斜率法、改良最大斜率法、去卷积算法分别测量肾皮质灌注参数，并以去卷积算法为标准评价最大斜率法、改良最大斜率法的准确性。结果显示，最大斜率法在低注射流率下会低估组织的血流量（Blood flow，BF），注射流率越低，低估的程度越高。改良最大斜率法与去卷积算法所得结果差异无显著性意义。下面我们对该内容进行详细介绍。

1 资料与方法

40例健康成人（男20例，女20例）随机等分为2组，行双肾皮质 CT 灌注扫描，一组注射流率为4 ml/s，另一组为2 ml/s，对比剂为优维显，用量为40 ml。CT 机型为 Siemens Somatom Plus 4，扫描序列为 Body perfusion，准直器宽度为5 mm，120 kV，300 mAs，层厚为10 mm，定位在肾门水平，扫描周期为1 s，每例扫40次，延迟6 s，屏气扫描。分别在腹主动脉（代替肾动脉）及肾皮质内画兴趣区，画兴趣区时注意与脏器边缘保持适当距离，以减少部分容积效应的影响，在此前提下争取尽可能大的面积以提高信噪比（图1）。把所得数据分别用去卷积算法、最大斜率法、改良最大斜率法（公式4）进行处理得出 BF。在相同注射流率下，对三种算法所得结果进行方差分析，两两比较采用最小显著差异（least significant difference，LSD）t 检验。考虑本研究样本含量较小，个体间的差异对两个不同注射流率组所得结果的影响较大，所以没有进行不同注射流率组间的比较。

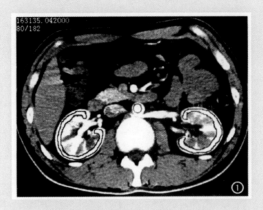

图1　双肾皮质感兴趣区的绘制

2　结果

注射流率为 4 ml/s 组不同算法所得血流灌注值及其统计处理结果见表1。模型 F =
9.15，P =0.0004。去卷积算法和改良最大斜率法所得血流灌注值分别为（4.20 ±
0.42）ml/（min·ml）、（4.10 ±0.53）ml/（min·ml），差异无显著性意义，两者很
接近，都高于最大斜率法的（3.60 ±0.47）ml/（min·ml）。以去卷积算法为标准，
最大斜率法对组织的血流灌注低估了约14 %。注射流率为 2 ml/s 组不同算法所得血流
灌注值及其统计处理结果见表2，模型 F =22.52，P <0.0001。同样去卷积算法和改良
最大斜率法所得血流灌注值分别为（4.35 ± 0.54）ml/（min·ml）和（4.28 ±
0.56）ml/（min·ml），差异无显著性意义，两者也很接近，都高于最大斜率法（3.35
±0.48）ml/（min ml）。以去卷积算法为标准，最大斜率法对组织的血流灌注低估了
约23 %。

表1　4 ml/s 注射组血流灌注值

统计值	去卷积算法	最大斜率法	改良最大斜率法
均数	4.20	3.60	4.10
标准差	0.42	0.47	0.53
95% 可信区间上限	4.00	3.38	3.85
95% 可信区间下限	4.40	3.82	4.35
t 检验（LSD）*	A	B	A

注：相同字母表示差异无显著性意义，反之为差异有显著性意义，检验水准 α =0.05

表2　2 ml/s 注射组血流灌注值

统计值	去卷积算法	最大斜率法	改良最大斜率法
均数	4.35	3.35	4.28
标准差	0.54	0.48	0.56
95%可信区间上限	4.10	3.12	4.02
95%可信区间下限	4.60	3.58	4.54
t 检验（LSD）*	A	B	A

注：相同字母表示差异无显著性意义，反之为差异有显著性意义，检验水准 α = 0.05

　　理论和实践都已证明，在对比剂的注射流率低于 10 ml/s 时用最大斜率法进行组织灌注测量，会产生对灌注值的低估，而且注射流率越低，低估的程度会越大。本研究采用的改良最大斜率法在低流率注射条件下可以计算出较为准确的组织血流灌注值（与去卷积算法所得结果一致），同时还具有采集数据少、扫描时间短（包括组织增强 TDC 的上升段即可）、计算简便的特点，适合临床常用注射流率下 CT 组织灌注值的近似计算。改良最大斜率法扩大了最大斜率法的适用范围，可适用于血管条件较差的受检者（血管纤细、弹性差、易破裂等），同时减少了因为对比剂注射流率过高给受检者带来的危险。

参考文献

［1］ Yoshiharu Ohno, Hisanobu Koyama, Ho Yun Lee, et al. Contrast - enhanced CT - and MRI - based perfusion assessment for pulmonary diseases： basics and clinical applications ［J］. Diagn Interv Radiol, DOI 10. 5152/dir. 2016, 161： 23.

［2］ Schoepf UJ, Bruening R, Konschitzky H, et al. Pulmonary embolism： comprehensive diagnosis by using electron - beam CT for detection of emboli and assessment of pulmonary blood flow ［J］. Radiology, 2000, 217： 693 - 700.

［3］ Hoffman EA, Chon D. Computed tomography studies of lung ventilation and perfusion ［J］. Proc Am Thorac Soc, 2005, 2： 492 - 498.

［4］ Ng QS, Goh V, Fichte H, et al. Lung cancer perfusion at multi - detector row CT： reproducibility of whole tumor quantitative measurements ［J］. Radiology, 2006, 239： 547 - 553.

［5］ Sitartchouk I, Roberts HC, Pereira AM, et al. Computed tomography perfusion using first pass methods for lung nodule characterization ［J］. Invest Radiol, 2008, 43： 349 - 358.

［6］ Wang J, Wu N, Cham MD, Song Y. Tumor response in patients with advanced non - small cell lung cancer： perfusion CT evaluation of chemotherapy and radiation therapy ［J］. Am J Roentgenol, 2009, 193： 1090 - 1096.

［7］ Li Y, Yang ZG, Chen TW, Yu JQ, et al. First - pass perfusion imaging of solitary pulmonary nodules with 64 - detector row CT： comparison of perfusion parameters of malignant and benign lesions ［J］. Br J Radiol, 2010, 83： 785 - 790.

［8］　Traupe H, Heiss WD, Hoeffken W, et al. Hyperperfusion and enhancement in dynamic computed tomography of ischemic stroke patients ［J］. J Comput Assist Tomogr, 1979, 3 (5)：627 – 632.

［9］　Miles KA. Measurement of tissue perfusion by dynamic computed tomography ［J］. Br J Radiol, 1991, 64 (761)：409 – 412.

［10］　Axel L. Tissue mean transit time from dynamic computed tomography by a simple deconvolution technique ［J］. Invest Radiol, 1983, 18 (1)：94 – 99.

［11］　Eastwood JD, Lev MH, Azhari T, et al. CT perfusion scanning with deconvolution analysis：pilot study in patients with acute middle cerebral artery stroke ［J］. Radiology, 2002, 222 (1)：227 – 236.

［12］　Hindmarsh T. Elimination of water – soluble contrast media from the subarachnoid space. Investigation with computer tomography ［J］. Acta Radiol Suppl, 1975, 346：45 – 49.

［13］　袁小东，张静，田建明，等. CT 灌注测量中去卷积算法准确性的检验 ［J］. 中国医学影像技术, 2005, 21 (5)：802 – 805.

［14］　Cuenod CA, Leconte I, Siauve N, et al. Deconvolution technique for measuring tissue perfusion by dynamic CT：application to normal and metastatic liver ［J］. Acad Radiol, 2002, 9 (Suppl 1)：S205 – 211.

［15］　Silverman M, Burgen AS. Application of analogue computer to measurement of intestinal absorption rates with tracers ［J］. J Appl Physiol, 1961, 16：911 – 913.

［16］　Langenbucher F. Handling of computational in vitro/in vivo correlation problems by Microsoft Excel：V. Predictive absorbability models ［J］. Eur J Pharm Biopharm. 2007, 67 (1)：293 – 299.

［17］　Langenbucher F. Handling of computational in vitro/in vivo correlation problems by Microsoft Excel：Ⅲ Convolution and deconvolution ［J］. Eur J Pharm Biopharm, 2003, 56 (3)：429 – 437.

［18］　袁小东，张静，田建明，等. CT 灌注在低注射流率时最大斜率法的准确性分析及改良 ［J］. 放射学实践, 2005, 20 (4)：345 – 348.

第二章

肺部双重供血 CT 灌注技术原理

肺部结节样病灶（肺结节）发病率高，病理种类涵盖肿瘤、炎症、结核等众多肺部疾病。癌性结节和良性结节的治疗方法及预后差异悬殊：癌性结节需要早诊早治，常用手术和/或放、化疗等有损伤的治疗手段，部分患者由于发现和诊断不及时而丧失治疗时机；良性结节一般不需要采取有损伤的治疗方法，且预后良好，因此肺结节的定性诊断尤其重要。当前肺结节的筛查（发现）主要依靠胸片和胸透，然后通过 CT 初步定性，CT 鉴别困难时需行穿刺甚或手术切除病理活检来明确。由于良恶性结节的 CT 影像表现重叠较多，部分良性结节患者因此经受了不必要的肺部手术，而部分癌性结节因为被 CT 误判为良性而错失治疗时机。

血流灌注反映了组织的功能活动和代谢水平，组织发生病理改变时其血流动力学往往也会发生相应的变化以适应新的病理状态，常规 CT 检查主要依据病变的形态和密度变化推测其性质，CT 灌注检测在提供病变的形态、密度信息的同时还可以给出病变的血流动力学信息，反映病变的功能活动。如：超急性期脑梗死常规 CT 检查常无阳性发现，而灌注测量可以发现梗死区的血流量（BF）明显下降；癌组织因为生长代谢活跃往往比良性组织拥有更高的血流量。随着多层螺旋 CT 的出现及普及，CT 扫描的空间分辨力及时间分辨力大大提高，CT 灌注扫描变得越来越简单易行，在获得精细的解剖学信息的同时可以得到病变的血流动力学信息，全面分析病变性质，提高影像诊断的准确性。

第一节　肺双重供血 CT 灌注的理论基础

肺具有两套血管系统，即肺循环和体循环（也称支气管循环，血供主要起源于支气管动脉，也可来自肋间、胸廓内动脉等分支），生理状态下肺循环为肺实质提供主要的血流量，属功能性血管（摄入氧气排出二氧化碳），支气管循环主要营养各级支气管和肺的间质支持结构，属营养血管。尽管支气管循环仅占肺总血流量的很小部分（<5%），它在维持气道及肺功能方面发挥重要作用[1]，且病理条件下可塑性较强，诸多肺部疾病如肺癌、慢性阻塞性肺病等表现为支气管动脉（bronchial artery，BA）供血显著增加[1,2]。长期以来此两套循环系统对肺癌供血的百分组成一直未有定量的研究报道，支气管循环是否为肺癌的主要血供来源尚存在争议：大多数研究者认为肺癌主要由 BA 供血[2-5]，也有学者认为肺动脉（pulmonary artery，PA）也可能为肺癌的主要血供来源[6,7]。

CT 灌注测量是通过计算对比剂首次通过供血动脉及组织的两条时间密度曲线（time density curves，TDCs）得以实现的。既往肺部 CT 灌注使用单一血供模式（图 2-1-1）：当肺实质作为主要研究对象时，PA 主干往往作为灌注分析的输入动脉，因为它是肺实质的主要血供来源[9~11]；反之当肺癌作为研究对象时，胸主动脉（替代 BA）则被选择为输入动脉，因为 BA 常被认为是肺癌的主要血供来源[2,8]。单一血供 CT 灌注无法同时测量肺循环和体循环，也就不能明确肿瘤组织的主要血供来源和双循环供血的比例。CT 灌注由于能够反映肿瘤的微循环状态，和瘤血管的生成及瘤细胞的代谢高度相关，被许多研究者用来评价肿瘤的良恶性。利用 CT 灌注成像（单血供模式）评价肺结节一度成为该领域的研究热点（Ohno Y，Koyama H，Matsumoto K 等），但是结果并不如预期的那么理想，其诊断癌性结节的敏感度和特异度在 70%~80%，尚不能用于临床。可能原因是：肺癌接受体、肺双循环供血的血流动力学特征并不能为单血供 CT 灌注所反映。本书作者在 2011 年年底带来团队建立了肺部的双重供血 CT 灌注（dual–input CT perfusion，DI–CTP）技术[9]，随即便开始肺结节的灌注研究。前期小样本研究结果提示癌性结节主要由体循环供血，良性结节正好相反——主要由肺循环供血，这种差别有助于结节的定性诊断，但是需要更大样本的研究来证实这些发现，并最终把这项技术推向临床。

基于最大斜率法的双重供血 CT 灌注最早由 Miles[10] 提出并用来定量研究肝脏的门静脉和肝动脉（体循环）供血：以腹主动脉和门静脉作为输入血管（input artery），脾脏的峰值时间点为分界线（区分肝动脉循环和门静脉循环），采用最大斜率法得到肝脏两套循环的血流量和比例。肺与肝这两种脏器都具有两套供血系统和类似的血流动力学特征，因此肝脏的双循环 CT 灌注模式理论上可以移植到肺的灌注成像上。我们的前期研究受到 Miles 方法的启发，以肺动脉和胸主动脉同时作为输入动脉，以左心房强化峰值时间点作为分界线获得肺循环和支气管循环的量化值和灌注图（图 2–1–2，图 2–1–3），此项研究成果发表在 2012 年 European Radiology 第 8 期上[9]。

DI–CTP 能更真实地评估肺肿瘤的灌注信息，它以肺动脉和胸主动脉同时作为输入动脉，以左心房强化峰值时间点为分界线区分肺循环和支气管循环（图 2–1–2，图 2–1–3），并利用最大斜率法计算 PF，BF 及 PI[9,10]。

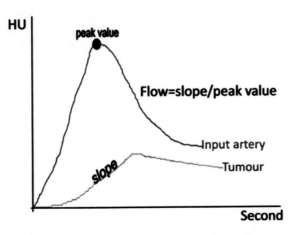

图 2–1–1　单血供 CT 灌注（最大斜率法）示意图
血流量等于肿瘤组织时间密度曲线（TDC）的最大斜率与主动脉强化峰值的比值

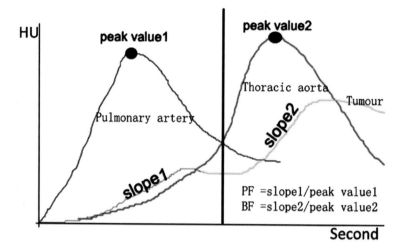

图 2-1-2 肺双血供 CT 灌注（DI-CTP，最大斜率法）示意图

肺动脉和胸主动脉同时作为供血血管，左心房增强的峰值时间点用于区分肺循环和支气管循环，以最大斜率法计算出两套循环的血流量

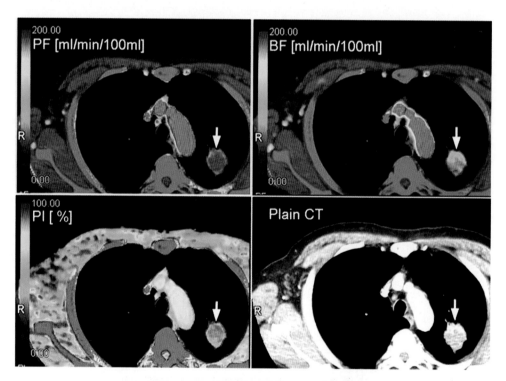

图 2-1-3 肺结节双重供血 CT 灌注图

结节位于左上肺，CT 灌注成像显示支气管动脉血流丰富（BF），肺动脉血流相对缺乏（PF），肺循环在总血流量中占的比例较小（PI），术后病理诊断为腺癌

第二节　肺双重供血 CT 灌注技术的实施细节

一、CT 容积肺灌注及测量

检查前所有患者都进行屏气训练，以确保其在整个灌注扫描过程中能屏住呼吸（约 30 s），如患者无法保持在整个 CT 数据采集期间屏住呼吸，允许在采集后期行浅式腹式呼吸。2 只 20G 静脉留置针分别置于两侧肘前静脉。采用 320 排 CT（Aquilion ONE，Toshiba Medical Systems，Otawara，Japan）行容积灌注扫描：电压 80 kV，电流 80 mA，扫描架旋转时间 0.5 s，迭代重建，重建层厚 0.5 mm，16 cm 探测器宽度覆盖病灶及肺门。灌注扫描前，先行整个胸部螺旋 CT 平扫用于确定肺内占位性病变的位置，之后采用高压注射器静脉注射 60 ml 370 mgI/ml 非离子型碘造影剂碘普罗胺（Bayer Schering，German），流率 8 ml/s（每侧 4 ml/s），团注后 2 s，扫描床不动，以 2 s 为间隔，进行 15 个低剂量容积采集（图 2-2-1）。在造影剂到达心脏前采集的最早两个容积数据作为基线，屏气时间约为 30 s，共生成 320×15＝4800 幅灌注图像。

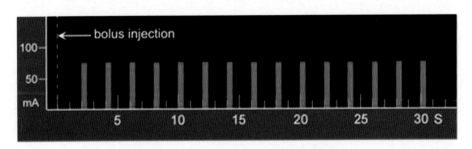

图 2-2-1　动态容积 CT 扫描流程图

二、后处理及灌注测量

每位患者图像重建约需 5 min。采用灌注软件（Dual-input Body Perfusion，Toshiba Medical Systems，Otawara，Japan）首先进行图像配准（registration）以消除体位移动或脏器活动引起的错位，并创建一个配准的容积序列，然后加载到体部灌注分析软件中。然后在肺门水平的肺动脉主干、降主动脉及肺结节灶内手工绘制感兴趣区（Region of interesting，ROI）以生成 3 条 TDC 曲线，分别代表 PA 循环输入函数、BA 循环输入函数及对比剂首次通过组织的反应函数（图 2-1-2，2-1-3）。绘制 ROI 时血管内 ROI 为矩形，平均面积为 1.0 cm²，病灶内 ROI 为椭圆形。此外在左心房内也绘制 ROI 生成 TDC，其峰值时间用于区分肺循环（峰值时间前）和支气管循环（峰值时间后）。预先设置窗宽范围为 0~150 HU，以确保肺结节灶的灌注得到良好显示，最后运行灌注软件，自动生成灌注参数图（PF，BF，PI；512×512 矩阵彩色编码）（图 2-2-2）。

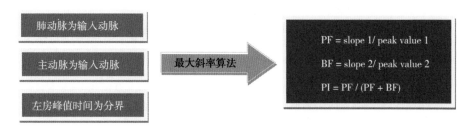

图 2 - 2 - 2　DI - CTP 示意图

CT 扫描辐射剂量计算参照 Valentin 等 2007 年在 Ann ICRP 公布的 DLP. e 乘以系数 0. 014 得出，我们的前期研究显示受检者人均辐射量在 3 ~ 4 mSv，相当于常规肝脏三期增强 CT 的辐射量，辐射剂量在临床能够接受的范围内。

三、DI - CTP 的临床应用价值

既往肺部 CT 灌注分析使用单入口灌注模型，选择肺动脉（pulmonary artery，PA）或主动脉（替代支气管动脉 bronchial artery，BA）作为供血动脉。关于肺部病灶特别是肺癌供血动脉的起源和/或血供比例一直有一些争议[2,11-14]。如果认为 BA 是肺癌唯一的或占主导地位的血供，就选择主动脉作为输入动脉；反之，如果认为 PA 是肺癌唯一的或占主导地位的血供，就选择肺动脉作为输入动脉。

早在 20 世纪 70 年代初，尸检研究发现肺肿瘤具有双重血管供应[15]；然而在活体内采用传统 MDCT 灌注技术定量肺癌双重血供在很大程度上由于技术的局限性较难实现。而了解肺肿瘤双套血供灌注定量参数和各自供血的相对比例信息可潜在有助于肺癌的治疗。本章介绍的 DI - CTP 技术是我们研究小组开发的一项 CT 灌注新技术，用于肺肿瘤的双重血供定量测量。该技术利用了超宽探测器 CT 获得肺部动态容积扫描数据，以肺动脉和胸主动脉为输入动脉，采用最大斜率算法行肺结节灌注评价，获得肺循环和体循环血流量（pulmonary flow，PF；bronchial flow，BF）及血流灌注指数［perfusion index，PI；PI = PF/（PF + BF）］。最大斜率法采用两个供血血管的 TDC 作为动脉输入函数来计算一个器官的双血供的概念，最初由 Miles 等人描述用于计算肝脏灌注[10]。腹主动脉和门静脉被选择作为双供血血管，脾脏增强的峰值时间点用来区分肝动脉循环和门静脉循环。根据最大斜率法，两个血管的血流量可通过组织增强的最大斜率除以两个供血动脉增强的峰值来获得[16]。同样在我们的技术应用中，PA 和 BA 分别被选择作为两输入血管，左心房的峰值增强时间点被用来区分肺循环和体循环。图 2 - 1 - 2 显示了这个时间点位于 PA 和 BA 的 TDCs 两峰之间，所以它是区分这两个循环之间的一个适当的分界点。当左心房没有被包括在 16 cm 的覆盖范围内时，可以手动设置两个峰之间的分界，理论上可获得相同的结果。考虑到左心房从功能上也正好是位于肺循环和支气管循环之间，因此其峰值强化时间点被选择用于划分组织的 TDC 为"肺循环部分"和"支气管循环部分"。然后由后处理软件分别确定"肺循环部分"和"支气管循环部分"的最大斜率，并计算出各自的血流量，这是本技术的关键点。在图 2 - 2 - 3 中，组织 TDC 上表现出明显的转折点，正好在左心房的高峰时间，从而支持我们选择使用左心房峰值时间是合理的。在前期纳入的小样本队列研究中，有些病例，组织 TDC 表现

出第 1 个斜坡与第 2 个斜坡之间存在一个平台，即两者间没有明显的转折点。这种情况下，左心房的增强峰值出现在平台期，可用于区分两种循环。当采用单一输入动脉的 CT 灌注技术用于肺癌灌注分析时，根据最大斜率法理论，占主导地位的循环将被计算和忽略次要循环。以图 2 - 2 - 3 为例，斜率 2 被视为肿瘤的循环，而斜率 1 将被忽略。也就是说，关于肺癌灌注的结果，以往研究只是有效地测量了支气管循环，而整体上由于忽略了双血供从而低估了肺癌的灌注。

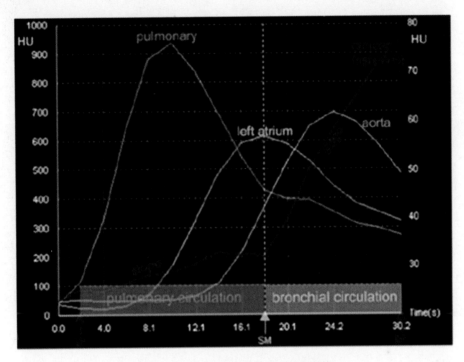

图 2 - 2 - 3　CT 灌注动态增强曲线图

上图为肺动脉（pulmonary）、主动脉（aorta）、左心房（left atrium）及肺癌（cancer）的时间密度曲线（time - density curves, TDCs）。图中纵向虚线代表了左心房强化的峰值时间点，它位于肺动脉 TDC 的下降段和主动脉 TDC 的上升段交汇处附近，因此该峰值时间点被用来分界肺循环和体循环，该时间点之前肺部病灶的灌注计算为肺循环血流量，该时间点之后病灶的灌注计算为体循环血流量；此例肺癌 TDC 的肺循环阶段呈缓慢上升，而体循环阶段呈急速上升，提示癌灶同时接受肺循环和体循环供血，且体循环血流量较大，是优势血供

　　DI - CTP 基于最大斜率法，仅考虑组织 TDC 初始斜坡和输入血管的增强峰值。因此，采集时间可短于去卷积算法分析，后者需要利用 TDC 的上升和下降部分。更短的采集时间使辐射剂量减低。然而，最大斜率分析方法也存在以下局限性：①血容量（blood volume, BV）、平均通过时间（mean transit time, MTT）不能直接采用最大斜率法生成；②对比剂通过双侧肘前静脉注射达到较高的流率，满足灌注模型假设要求。最大斜率法由于其理论假设组织最大增强要在静脉引流开始前出现，因此要求对比剂注射速率在 5 ~ 10 ml/s。在总对比剂量固定的情况下，更高的注射速率意味着更短的注射时间，会使得两输入动脉的 TDCS 坡度更陡峭，因此这个循环之间重叠区域会减少（图 2 - 2 - 4，图 2 - 2 - 5）[17]。重叠区域较大会在一定程度上削弱 DI - CTP 测量的可靠性，特别是肺循环残余灌注会影响体循环的评

价。此外，高注射流率可使组织增强最大化，并提高信噪比[18]。

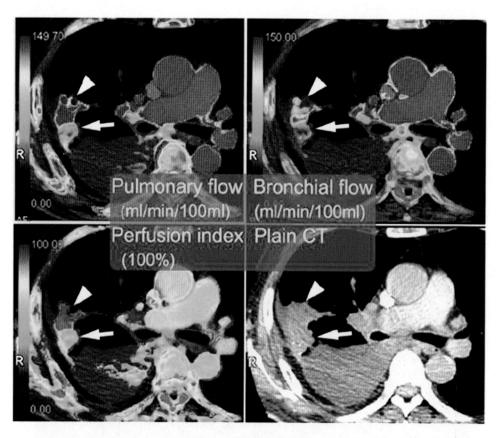

图 2 - 2 - 4　CT 灌注图

45 岁男性患者，病理证实为右下肺腺癌（箭），癌灶表现为相对丰富的肺动脉血流和支气管动脉血流，
相邻肺不张（箭头）表现为丰富的肺动脉血流和较弱的支气管动脉血流

在 320 排 CT 出现之前，从未有研究进行肺癌肿瘤组织的肺循环和支气管循环的同步评
估，主要是由于之前的设备沿 Z 轴方向的覆盖范围有限。Aquilion One 这一机型可行 16 cm
容积成像，沿 Z 轴方向可较容易覆盖成人肺的一半以上范围。肺门及病变通常可在一次成
像容积内包括。因此，PA、主动脉、左心房与病变的研究可在一次采集同时包括，使肺肿
瘤的 DICTP 分析成为可能。灌注 CT 的一个内在的限制是辐射暴露，这与管电压、管电流和
CT 容积采集的数量增加有关。为使 CT 辐射剂量控制在临床应用的范围内，我们降低了灌
注 CT 的 kV 和 mA，确保全部剂量（包括定位成像）约等于腹部三期扫描成像的剂量[19,20]。
此外，由于采集时间较短，我们利用最大斜率法而不是去卷积算法来计算灌注，因此可确保
我们的灌注扫描协议的目标剂量。容积 DICTP 后处理需要 5 ~ 10 min 校准。目前，该技术可
能还不太适合紧急病例。

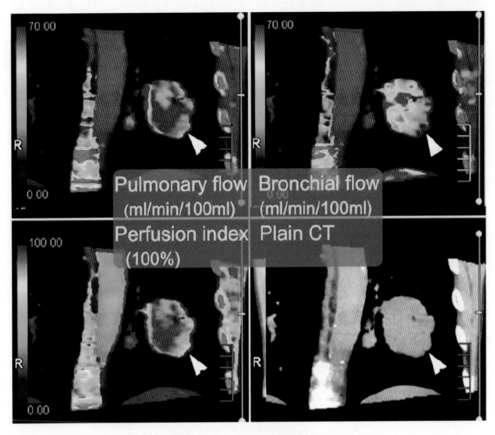

图 2 - 2 - 5　CT 灌注图冠状面

53 岁男性患者，病理证实为左下肺鳞状细胞癌，整个肿瘤呈不均匀灌注，肿瘤的外周区域主要由肺动脉供血（箭头）

参考文献

［1］ McCullagh A, Rosenthal M, Wanner A, et al. The bronchial circulation—worth a closer look: a review of the relationship between the bronchial vasculature and airway inflammation ［J］. Pediatr Pulmonol, 2010, 45: 1 - 13.

［2］ Hellekant C. Bronchial angiography and intraarterial chemotherapy with mitomycin—C in bronchogenic carcinoma: anatomy, technique, complications ［J］. Acta Radiol Diagn (Stockh), 1979, 20: 478 - 496.

［3］ Park HS, Kim YI, Kim HY, et al. Bronchial artery and systemic artery embolization in the management of primary lung cancer patients with hemoptysis ［J］. Cardiovasc Intervent Radiol, 2007, 30: 638 - 643.

［4］ Littleton JT, Durizch ML, Moeller G, et al. Pulmonary masses: contrast enhancement ［J］. Radiology, 1990, 177: 861 - 871.

［5］ Han MJ, Feng GS, Yang JY, et al. The pulmonary artery doesn't participate in the blood supply of lung cancer: experimental and DSA study ［J］. Chin J Radiol, 2000, 34: 802 - 804.

［6］ Botenga AS. The significance of broncho—pulmonary anastomoses in pulmonary anamolies: a selective angiographic study ［J］. Radiol Clin Biol, 1969, 38: 309 - 328.

[7] Pump KK. Distribution of bronchial arteries in the human lung [J]. Chest, 1972, 62: 447 – 451.

[8] Viamonte M Jr. Angiographic evaluation of lung neoplasms [J]. Radiol Clin North Am, 1965, 3: 529 – 542.

[9] Yuan XD, Zhang J, Ao GK. Lung cancer perfusion: can we measure pulmonary and bronchial circulation simultaneously [J]? Euro Radiol, 2012, 22 (8): 1665 – 1671.

[10] Miles KA, Hayball MP, Dixon AK. Functional images of hepatic perfusion obtained with dynamic CT [J]. Radiology, 1993, 188: 405 – 411.

[11] Tacelli N, Remy – Jardin M, Copin MC, et al. Assessment of non – small cell lung cancer perfusion: pathologic – CT correlation in 15 patients [J]. Radiology, 2010, 257: 863 – 871.

[12] Milne EN, Zerhouni AE. Blood supply of pulmonary metastases [J]. J Thoracic Imaging, 1987, 2: 15 – 23.

[13] Kiessling F, Boese J, Corvinus C, et al. Perfusion CTin patients with advanced bronchial carcinomas: a novel chance for characterization and treatment monitoring [J]? Eur Radiol, 2004, 14: 1226 – 1233.

[14] Viamonte M Jr. Angiographic evaluation of lung neoplasms [J]. Radiol Clin North Am, 1965, 3: 529 – 542.

[15] Milne EN. Circulation of primary and metastatic pulmonary neoplasms: a postmortem microarteriographic study [J]. Am J Roentgenol Radium Ther Nucl Med, 1967, 100: 603 – 619.

[16] Miles KA, Griffiths MR. Perfusion CT: a worthwhile enhancement [J]? Br J Radiol, 2003, 76: 220 – 231.

[17] Bae KT. Peak contrast enhancement in CT and MR angiography: when does it occur and why? Pharmacokinetic study in a porcine model [J]. Radiology, 2003, 227: 809 – 816.

[18] Miles KA. Perfusion CT for the assessment of tumour vascularity: which protocol [J]? Br J Radiol, 2003, 76: S36 – S42.

[19] Galanski M, Nagel HD, Stamm G. Results of a federation inquiry 2005/2006: pediatric CT X – ray practice in Germany [J]. Rofo, 2007, 179: 1110 – 1111.

[20] Tsai HY, Tung CJ, Yu CC, et al. Survey of computed tomography scanners in Taiwan: dose descriptors, dose guidance levels, and effective doses [J]. Med Phys, 2007, 34: 1234 – 1243.

第三章

肺部双重供血 CT 灌注技术临床研究

第一节　肺部双重供血 CT 灌注技术对
肺良恶性孤立性肺结节的判别价值

早在 20 世纪 70 年代初，研究人员就通过尸体微动脉造影成像发现肺部肿瘤具有双套血液供应，即肺循环和体循环[1]。肺部肿瘤病理类型不同，两套血液循环供应比例（即灌注）也是不同的，了解病灶血供特点对病变定性及治疗方案的选择均具有重要的意义。既往由于 MDCT 探测器宽度及胸部 Z 轴覆盖范围有限，在大多数情况下，只能选择主动脉作为输入动脉，而肺动脉通常不能被包含成像区域内，因此评估肺肿瘤的血流动力学参数只能采用单血供灌注模型，无法进行双重供血的灌注定量方法测量。320 排 CT 设备的临床应用，有效地解决了上述问题，其可以提供更大的 Z 轴覆盖范围，使得活体内肺癌双血供的 CT 灌注定量成为可能[2]。利用 320 排 CT 动态容积扫描模式，检查床不动，机架单次旋转，即可实现胸部 16 cm 的覆盖范围，同时包括肺动脉、主动脉和肺部病灶，之后对比剂增强的动态容积数据采集同步获得体循环和肺循环的动脉输入函数以及肺部病灶组织的首过反应函数。

孤立性结节（solitary pulmonary nodule，SPN）是肺内单发直径 ≤3 cm 的完全被肺实质所包围的圆形或类圆形病灶，不伴有明显的肺不张、炎症或局部淋巴结肿大。由于孤立性肺结节影像征象复杂多样，定性较为困难。准确识别恶性肺结节并有效地制订治疗策略能显著降低肺部恶性肿瘤的死亡率[3]。一直以来，放射科医生面对的主要挑战是肺的孤立性良、恶性结节在常规 CT 上形态学方面存在巨大的重叠。随着多排螺旋 CT 设备及 CT 灌注成像技术的发展，灌注测量生成的血流动力学参数用以帮助识别肺癌[4,5]。采用最大斜率算法的单供血分析模型在一定程度上可用于此目的，并被证明可帮助恶性和良性结节的鉴别[6,7]。理论上，不同性质的 SPNs 具有不同比例的肺循环和体循环供血，是否更有可能帮助鉴别肺癌？在 2011~2012 年间本研究小组采用前瞻性设计，研究了 DI – CTP 在识别良、恶性孤立性肺结节的价值。

该研究连续纳入了 56 例 SPNs 患者（31 名男性，25 名女性，平均年龄 51 岁，范围37~66 岁）。所有患者均在 CT 灌注扫描之前或之后 2 周内经 CT 引导下穿刺活检或纤支镜活检或手术切除获得病理结果，包括 32 例恶性 SPNs：鳞癌 11 例，腺鳞癌 6 例，腺癌 11 例，小细胞肺癌 4 例；24 例良性 SPNs：7 例炎性假瘤，8 例结核瘤，4 例错构瘤，4 例球形肺炎，1 例硬化性血管瘤。肿瘤平均大小为 10.7 cm³（2.4~44.1 cm³）。所有患者均进行了上一章节介绍的 DI – CTP 灌注成像（扫描细节及后处理方法同前）。

CT灌注扫描过程中，尽管对比剂注射速率相对较高，且要求屏气持续时间为30 s相对较长，但所有患者均表现出良好的依从性，没有发生严重的不良事件。11例患者在扫描末期因缺氧而采取浅腹式呼吸。灌注参数图采用可视化的伪彩图显示，并与原始轴位CT图像融合。代表性的灌注彩色图如图3 - 1 - 1、3 - 1 - 2所示。56例SPNs的DI - CTP灌注结果列于表3 - 1 - 1和图3 - 1 - 3。良、恶性肿瘤的三个灌注参数在两者间均存在显著的统计学差异，其中PI的差别最大：恶性为0.30 ± 0.07，良性为0.51 ± 0.13，P < 0.001。PI的ROC下面积为0.92，为三个灌注参数中最大，识别肺癌的敏感度为0.95，特异度为0.83，+ LR为5.59，- LR为0.06。

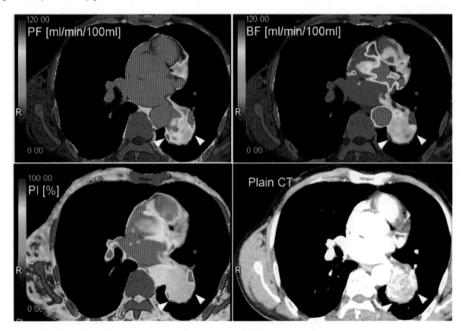

图3 - 1 - 1 横断面灌注图

左下肺肿块同时接受肺循环和体循环血供，两者均较丰富，以肺动脉血流略占优势，病理结果为炎性假瘤

表3 - 1 - 1 灌注参数及ROC分析结果

灌注参数	例数	均数	标准差	95% CI Lower	95% CI Upper	t检验	ROC面积 (95% CI)
PF（ml/min/100 ml）							
恶性	32	24.56	10.85	20.65	28.47	P < 0.001	0.85
良性	24	44.88	16.01	38.12	51.64		(0.75 ~ 0.96)
BF（ml/min/100 ml）							
恶性	32	58.17	26.78	48.51	67.82	P = 0.028	0.66
良性	24	43.32	20.56	34.64	52.00		(0.52 ~ 0.81)
PI（100%）							
恶性	32	0.30	0.07	0.27	0.33	P < 0.001	0.92
良性	24	0.51	0.13	0.46	0.57		(0.85 ~ 1.00)

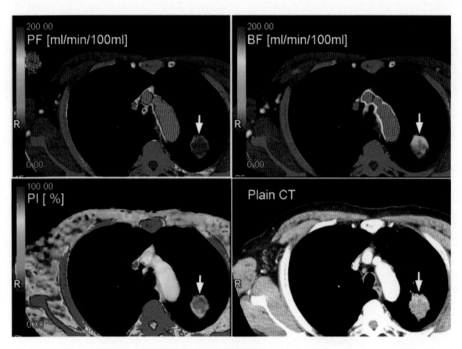

图 3 - 1 - 2　横断面灌注图

左上肺肿块具有较丰富的体循环供血（支气管动脉供血），基本没有肺动脉血供，病理结果为腺癌

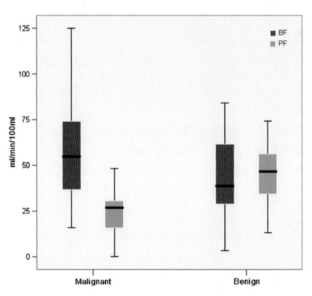

图 3 - 1 - 3　恶性肿瘤往往支气管动脉血供占优势，而肺部的良性病灶的支气管动脉血供无此优势

肺灌注与肝脏灌注类似，肺脏与肝脏的血管系统无论从解剖学还是功能学角度来讲都非常接近，都具有双套供血系统并具有相似的血流动力学特征。自 Miles 等首次报道 CT 双入口灌注 (dual-input CT perfusion，DICTp) 模型以来，其在肝灌注中的应用得到普遍认可，因此有理由相信这种模型在肺灌注中也是可行的。直到 320 排 CT 出现之后，肺癌的两种供血血流测量成为可能。肺癌存在支气管动脉的血流供应已通过支气管动脉血管造影等研究[9]证实。另一方面，有关活体内肺癌存在肺循环供血的研究报道很少，仅有先前的一项研究[10]提示，一些肺癌病灶的增强早于主动脉的增强，反映了存在肺动脉供应的血流。理论上，单供血最大斜率算法采用组织 TDC 的最大斜率与供血动脉 TDC 上 CT 值最大峰值之比计算血流量，在双循环系统的情况下，如肺和支气管循环，组织 TDC 最大斜率只是代表了占主导供血地位的血流量，而次要血供的血流量就会被忽略。考虑到肺癌的支气管或体循环动脉血流量相对高于肺动脉的血流量 (图 3-1-2，图 3-1-3)，单供血最大斜率算法分析结果只是支气管动脉的血流。反之亦然，良性肿瘤的分析结果反映的是肺动脉的血流量。继往 CT 灌注在肺癌诊断方面的价值之所以同本研究所体现的不同，主要的原因可能是继往 CT 灌注对肿瘤的血供评价并不全面[11]。本项研究中，所有病灶内两种循环血流比例是异质性分布的 (图 3-1-2)；局部区域测量与肿瘤整体测量显著不同。这也可能是本研究和以前报道的研究之间的差异的另一个原因，继往 CT 设备由于有限的探测器宽度，CT 灌注测量仅能在病灶有限的一或两层 CT 断面进行。就正常肺组织的总血流量而言，支气管动脉血流分数非常低，为 1%~2%。然而，支气管动脉血流对于维持气道和肺功能是至关重要的[12]，特别是在病理条件下，其具有极强的可塑性。在肺癌中，支气管动脉血流就会增加。本项研究结果支持在恶性 SPNs 病灶中，支气管动脉血流量非常显著，而肺动脉血流量相对较低 (表 3-1-1，图 3-1-2，图 3-1-3)，恶性 SPNs 中肺动脉指数 PI 仅为 0.30 ± 0.07。而在良性肿瘤中，肺循环和支气管循环的比例几近平衡，PI 为 0.51 ± 0.13。这些研究结果不仅有利于肺癌的鉴别诊断，而且有助于肺癌治疗计划的制订：①如果肺癌患者需行介入治疗，临床医生就可以根据 DI-CTP 结果中的 PI 制订决策，即是经肺动脉还是经支气管动脉治疗；②由于肺循环和体循环中血氧浓度不同，PI 提示了 BA 的灌注比例，反映了肿瘤中的氧饱和度。据报道，高水平的血氧会导致肿瘤对放疗的敏感性[13]。因此 PI 在肺癌放疗的疗效预测中具有潜在的应用价值。

受试者工作特性曲线分析是用来评估某一参数对特定疾病的诊断表现，该曲线下的面积反映了该参数的诊断效能：面积越大，诊断效能越高[14]。本研究的三个灌注参数 ROC 曲线中，PI 具有最大的 ROC 面积，表明 PI 区分恶性和良性 SPNs 的诊断效能最高 (图 3-1-4)。为了进一步确定其灵敏度和特异度，曲线上的一个临界值点需要被确定。通常这一点位于最靠近 ROC 坐标系的左上角。本研究中 PI 的临界值是 0.42，对应地敏感度为 0.95，特异性为 0.83，+LR 5.59，-LR 0.06。阳性和阴性预测值 (PPV 和 NPV) 在一组患者中确认和排除恶性肿瘤的诊断取决于研究队列中恶性肿瘤的患病率。相比之下，-LR 和 +LR 在界定恶性肿瘤的诊断效率方面被视为比 PPV 和 NPV 更稳定，因此被选择用于本研究[15,16]。当 +LR > 10，-LR < 0.1，就有足够的信心去确认或排除某些疾病。对应的，如果一例 SPNs 的 PI 值高于 0.42，肺癌的诊断就有足够信心可以排除；而如果 PI 值低于 0.42，由于较低的 +LR (5.59)，只能是提示有肺癌诊断的可能，但信心不足，。进一步可采用如活检等手段来确认诊断。

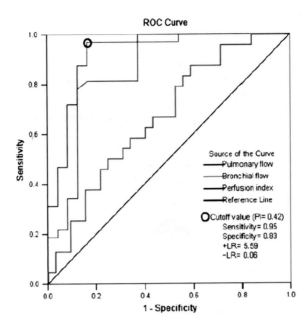

图 3 - 1 - 4　受试者工作特性曲线（receiver - operating characteristic，ROC）
分析显示：灌注指数对鉴别肺部病灶的良恶性有帮助，支气管动脉血供占优势可能提示病灶为恶性，支气管动脉血供和肺动脉血供水平相当或肺动脉血供占优势者为良性病灶的可能性大一些

　　本项研究的局限性：首先，这两种循环的重叠可能会削弱灌注测量的有效性。采用通过左右两肘前静脉高的对比剂注射速率以及因此导致注射持续时间缩短会减少这种重叠（图 3 - 1 - 5）[2]。其次，本研究推荐采用 CT 原始解剖图和灌注参数图信息的整合（图像融合），比单独使用灌注测量在鉴别诊断方面更有帮助[17]，但是 CT 形态学和功能学信息整合的有效性需要进一步评估。再次，考虑到肺肿瘤病理类型的多样性和各种病理状态下血流动力学的不同，本研究中样本量相对较小，难免会导致选择性偏倚，可能在一定程度上会存在结果的偏倚。因此，基于人群的调查是必要的，以进一步确定本研究结果的临床价值。最后，辐射暴露是灌注 CT 固有的局限，其需要增加管电压、管电流和 CT 容积暴露的数量。为了维持整体辐射剂量在临床应用范围内，本研究降低了 CT 灌注的管电压和管电流，最终辐射剂量与腹部三期扫描剂量相当[18,19]。

　　总之，基于最大斜率法的 DI - CTP 得到的 PI 能代表 SPNs 病灶中肺循环在两套循环中的灌注比例，是鉴别恶性与良性孤立性肺结节的一个非常有价值的生物标志物。灌注指数对肺癌治疗计划的制订以及放疗疗效的预测也具有潜在的应用价值。

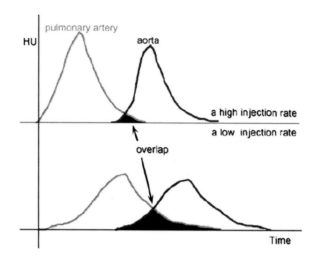

图 3 - 1 - 5　在对比剂用量固定的情况下，注射流率越大，肺循环和体循环在时相上的重叠越少，双重供血的灌注测量越精确；反之，注射流率越小，两个循环之间的重叠越多，测量结果越不可靠

参考文献

［1］　Milne EN. Circulation of primary and metastatic pulmonary neoplasms：a postmortem microarteriographic study ［J］. Am J Roentgenol Radium Ther Nucl Med，1967，100：603 - 619.

［2］　Yuan X，Zhang J，Ao G，et al. Lung cancer perfusion：can we measure pulmonary and bronchial circulation simultaneously ［J］？ Eur Radiol，2010，22：1665 - 1671.

［3］　Nair A，Hansell DM. European and North American lung cancer screening experience and implications for pulmonary nodule management ［J］. Eur Radiol，2011，21：2445 - 2454.

［4］　Sitartchouk I，Roberts HC，Pereira AM，et al. Computed tomography perfusion using first pass methods for lung nodule characterization ［J］. Invest Radiol，2008，43：349 - 358.

［5］　Li Y，Yang ZG，Chen TW，et al. First - pass perfusion imaging of solitary pulmonary nodules with 64 - detector row CT：comparison of perfusion parameters of malignant and benign lesions ［J］. Br J Radiol，2010，83：785 - 790.

［6］　Zhang M，Kono M. Solitary pulmonary nodules：evaluation of blood flow patterns with dynamic CT ［J］. Radiology，1997，205：471 - 478.

［7］　Lee YH，Kwon W，Kim MS，et al. Lung perfusion CT：the differentiation of cavitary mass ［J］. Eur J Radiol，2010，73：59 - 65.

［8］　Valentin J. Managing patient dose in multi - detector computed tomography（MDCT）［J］. Ann ICRP，2007，37：1 - 79.

［9］　Luo L，Wang H，Ma H，et al. Analysis of 41 cases of primary hypervascular non - small cell lung cancer treated with embolization of emulsion of chemotherapeutics and iodized oil ［J］. Zhongguo Fei Ai Za Zhi，2010，13：540 - 543.

［10］　Kiessling F，Boese J，Corvinus C. Perfusion CT in patients with advanced bronchial carcinomas：a novel chance for characterization and treatment monitoring [J]? Eur Radiol, 2004, 14: 1226 – 1233.

[11] Ohno Y, Koyama H, Matsumoto K, et al. Differentiation of malignant and benign pulmonary nodules with quantitative first – pass 320 – detector row perfusion CT versus FDG PET/CT [J]. Radiology, 2011, 258: 599 – 609.

[12] McCullagh A, Rosenthal M, Wanner A, et al. The bronchial circulation – worth a closer look: a review of the relationship between the bronchial vasculature and airway inflammation [J]. Pediatr Pulmonol, 2010, 45: 1 – 13.

[13] Wang J, Ning W, Cham MD, et al. Tumor response in patients with advanced non – small cell lung cancer: perfusion CT evaluation of chemotherapy and radiation therapy [J]. Am J Roentgenol, 2009, 193: 1090 – 1096.

[14] He H, Lyness JM, McDermott MP. Direct estimation of the area under the receiver operating characteristic curve in the presence of verification bias [J]. Stat Med, 2009, 28: 361 – 376.

[15] Goehring C, Perrier A, Morabia A. Spectrum bias: a quantitative and graphical analysis of the variability of medical diagnostic test performance [J]. Stat Med, 2004, 23: 125 – 135.

[16] Bhandari M, Guyatt GH. How to appraise a diagnostic test [J]. World J Surg, 2005, 29: 561 – 566.

[17] Marten K, Grabbe E. The challenge of the solitary pulmonary nodule: diagnostic assessment with multislice spiral CT [J]. Clin Imaging, 2003, 27: 156 – 161.

[18] Tsai HY, Tung CJ, Yu CC, et al. Survey of computed tomography scanners in Taiwan: dose descriptors, dose guidance levels, and effective doses [J]. Med Phys, 2007, 34: 1234 – 1243.

[19] Galanski M, Nagel HD, Stamm G. Results of a federation inquiry 2005/2006: pediatric CT X – ray practice in Germany [J]. Rofo, 2007, 179: 1110 – 1111.

第二节 肺部双重供血 CT 灌注技术对肺结核及结核伴发体循环动脉—肺动脉瘘的诊断价值

近年来肺结核的发病率逐年增高，肺结核治疗后耐药也成了临床上比较棘手的问题。此外，咯血也是肺结核常见的并发症之一，急性大咯血保守治疗效果不佳，易复发且病死率较高。MDCT 检查可明确结核病灶并通过肺组织内积血判断出血部位，但无法对结核病灶造成的血管损伤进行检测和评估，只有在动脉栓塞介入治疗时数字减影血管造影（DSA）才可发现异常出血动脉。体循环动脉肺动脉瘘简称"体肺动脉瘘"，为最常见的间接出血征象，320 层肺双血供 CT 灌注技术的临床应用，为检测体肺动脉瘘提供了可能。

通过前述章节的分析，单血供 CT 灌注技术仅能分析肺及肺部病灶主要供血的灌注情况，不能完全胜任于双血供特征的研究；此外，目前针对肺结核等肺部其他疾病的在体血流动力学研究也相对较少，考虑到血流动力学特征对病变的发生、发展、诊断、治疗及随访预后等诸多方面潜在的影响，本研究小组在 2011—2016 年间应用 DICTP 技术研究了肺结核活动性病灶的血流动力学特征，并通过肺结核大咯血患者 DI – CTP 成像和 DSA 对比分析，探讨了 DI – CTP 检出和定位肺结核大咯血患者体肺动脉瘘的诊断价值[1,2]。此外，针对结核耐药问题，采用 DI – CTP 技术研究了复治涂阳肺结核病灶的血流动力学特征。

一、活动性肺结核病灶 DI – CTP 研究结果

本研究纳入了 25 例活动性肺结核患者（男 14 例，女 11 例，年龄 15～65 岁，平均 35

岁），临床诊断在灌注扫描前后 1 个月内通过针刺活检、纤维支气管镜检查或实验室及临床资料明确，CT 动态容积扫描及灌注扫描技术同前介绍，进行图像后处理时，也是在肺门水平的肺动脉主干、降主动脉及肺内病灶内手工绘制感兴趣区 ROIs 以生成 3 条 TDC 曲线，分别代表肺循环输入函数、体循环输入函数及组织的衰减函数，绘制 ROI 时血管内 ROI 为矩形，平均面积为 $1.0~cm^2$，病灶内 ROI 为手工绘制的自由形状贴合病灶的轮廓。此外，在左心房内也绘制 ROI 生成 TDC，其峰值时间用于区分肺循环（峰值时间前）和体循环（峰值时间后）。最后运行灌注软件，自动生成 512×512 矩阵编码的彩色图像，分别显示肺动脉血流量（pulmonary flow，PF）、支气管动脉血流量（bronchial flow，BF）及灌注指数［perfusion index，PI = PF/（PF + BF）］。

最终得到结核病灶灌注参数：PF（46.41±19.84）ml/min/100 ml，BF（20.91±11.98）ml/min/100 ml，PI 0.68±0.16；95% CI PF 为 38.22~54.60，BF 为 15.96~25.85，PF 为 0.62~0.75；PF 明显大于 BF，P<0.001。

本研究揭示肺部结核病灶接受肺循环和体循环双套血供，为支气管动脉—肺动脉瘘伴发于结核咯血提供了合理的解释：因为在结核病灶中同时存在两套血管系统，当病灶坏死后两套血管床亦有可能受破坏、相通，并在压力差的驱使下发生体动脉—肺动脉瘘；此外，本研究提示 PA 血流明显高于 BA 血流，暗示 PI 这一指标可能成为结核与肺癌相鉴别的有效标志，因为后者被大多数研究报道认为是 BA 供血占优势；另外，病灶血供的强弱还可用来判断结核病灶的活跃程度，通过治疗前后的对照监测疗效及指示预后。当然这些仅仅是合理推测，还需要相关的临床研究来进一步证实。

二、DI – CTP 应用于肺结核伴发体—肺动脉瘘的价值

约有 25% 的结核病患者在其病程中会发生咯血[3]。大咯血可危及患者生命，长期的临床诊疗实践证实结核性大咯血往往和肺内的体—肺动脉瘘密切相关，因此体—肺动脉瘘的明确诊断和对其有效的栓塞对结核性大咯血的治疗是至关重要的。为了进一步探讨 DI – CTP 技术在检出和定位肺结核伴体—肺动脉瘘的价值，我们连续纳入了 12 例肺结核大咯血患者，年龄 34~67 岁，平均年龄（47±16.3）岁；男 11 例，女 1 例。其中慢性纤维空洞性肺结核 4 例，陈旧性肺结核伴结核性支气管扩张 6 例，浸润性肺结核 2 例，病程为 6 个月至 30 余年。每日咯血量在 300~2000 ml，均为内科治疗无效而不能外科手术或不愿外科手术治疗的患者。

采用 320 层 CT 动态容积扫描及 DI – CTP 灌注扫描技术（同前），通过灌注软件完成后处理程序，得到相应的灌注参数图。

DI – CTP 检查后立即行 DSA 动脉造影及出血动脉栓塞治疗。采用 Seldinger 技术，将 5F Cobra 导管分别选择性双侧支气管动脉、肋间动脉和锁骨下动脉造影，分别采集 DSA 选择性动脉图像，观察体—肺动脉瘘，并和 DI – CTP 图像进行对比分析，判断瘘发生部位及肺动脉异常灌注肺段的显示。

所有患者均顺利地完成了灌注扫描，经过软件对位后，灌注图片无显著的移动伪影。本研究中 12 例患者共观察 216 个肺段全部纳入分析。依据 DSA 检查结果将各个肺段灌注参数分为有、无体—肺动脉瘘两组，检查发现存在循环动脉—肺动脉瘘肺段 70 个，阴性肺段

146 个，PF、BF 和 PI 在有和无体—肺动脉瘘存在的肺段灌注差异有统计学意义（三者 P 值均 <0.001）。在 PF、BF 和 PI 三个灌注参数中，PI 的 ROC 曲线下面积最大（P < 0.001），诊断效能最高，其诊断阈值为 96.25，敏感度 88.00%，特异度 87.00%。

CT 灌注成像技术能准确地显示组织的灌注状态且能进一步进行定量分析，使得组织内部血流动力学研究有了新的手段，而 DI－CTP 的应用使得肺灌注技术成功地将肺动脉和支气管动脉（体循环）的血流分别定量计算，从而使得体—肺动脉瘘得以清楚显示。本研究表明，PF、BF 和 PI 对体—肺动脉瘘的检出效能有所不同，PI 的 ROC 曲线下面积最大，提示 PI 的诊断效能最高，其诊断阈值为 96.25（ROC 曲线上最接近坐标左上角的点对应着阈值，该点的纵坐标与横坐标值分别对应着敏感度 88%、特异度 87%）。

肺结核咯血的原因及机制为：肺结核及其继发感染的细菌毒素及大量致敏物质使肺部局部出现炎性反应致肺毛细血管通透性增加，引起血细胞外渗入肺泡；干酪坏死造成病变组织坏死溶解而侵蚀破坏血管；诱发支气管扩张的发生，并伴发支气管循环血管的扭曲扩张，侧支循环增加，致使支气管和肺循环之间吻合增多，支气管壁黏膜破坏、糜烂、溃疡、肉芽组织毛细血管破坏出血[4]。传统的影像学诊断方法包括 X 线摄影、纤维支气管内镜、动脉造影、CT 等。DSA 一直以来被认为是金标准：DSA 血管造影可见支气管动脉及体循环侧支主干增粗、迂曲，病变区有大量新生血管和体—肺动脉瘘，常规血管造影可显示支气管动脉及体循环侧支和新生血管情况，但体—肺动脉瘘显示率不高[5-8]。

体－肺动脉瘘的血流动力改变和 CT 灌注特征可以做如下分析：①在肺动脉期由于瘘造成的体动脉—肺动脉分流，部分不含对比剂的体循环血液进入肺动脉与含对比剂的血液混合，因此在 PF 灌注图表现为低 PF 值肺段区域，在 ROC 曲线表现为相应峰值的下降；②在体循环期为含对比剂的体循环血液灌入，造成相应肺段区域的高灌注，而正常区域支气管动脉循环（体循环）仅占总血流量很小的一部分，造成了异常高灌注与正常灌注的较大反差，从而 BF 值增高；在 ROC 曲线表现为相应峰值的上升；③PI 值反映的是肺动脉在所有肺组织供血中的比例，由于 PF 峰值的下降和 BF 峰值的增高，使得 PI 值曲线下面积最大，临床意义最大。

本研究的局限性主要有两点：①纳入研究的患者数较少，相关结论尚需后续的大样本研究来支撑；②极少数结核性大咯血患者肺内表现为体—肺静脉瘘，不能为 DI－CTP 检出，还需要 DSA 进一步明确。

三、DI－CTP 技术用于评价复治涂阳肺结核病灶灌注特征的分析

结核病的耐药问题是结核病防治工作的难点，耐多药肺结核更可能成为不治之症。复治肺结核多由结核分枝杆菌耐药引起[9,10]，而细菌耐药的原因之一为长期低浓度的接触抗生素，因此，在关注有效血药浓度的同时观察病灶局部的微循环对病灶局部药物浓度的影响十分重要。应用 DI－CTP 技术即可定量评估病灶肺循环和体循环的血液灌注特征。

在 2015 年 5 月至 2016 年 1 月间，连续纳入经临床确诊的 54 例肺结核患者，其中结核球 6 例，浸润性病灶 21 例，空洞病灶 8 例，多形性病灶 19 例。根据治疗效果，分为初治治愈组 30 例、复治组 24 例［其中初治失败者 10 例（首次复治组），2 次及 2 次以上复治失败者 14 例（多次复治组）］，病程 3 个月至 15 年。入选患者均符合 2005 年中华医学会《临床

诊疗指南（结核病分册）》制定的复治失败肺结核的诊断标准[3]。复治患者：因结核病化疗方案不合理或不规律使用抗结核药物治疗≥1个月和/或初治失败和复发。痰菌检查：经痰抗酸杆菌涂片阳性和/或痰结核分枝杆菌培养阳性，经菌种鉴定排除非结核分枝杆菌。所有患者治疗后空腹血糖控制在 7.8 mmol/L 以下，无糖尿病眼底病变及糖尿病肾病。

所有患者均行 DI-CTP 技术扫描，方法同前。结果显示初治治愈组与复治组之间 PF（46.4±9.2 vs 25.9±7.6）、BF（18.9±10.0 vs 24.8±8.8）和 PI（0.6±0.2 vs 0.5±0.2）值均有统计学差异（P 值均<0.05）。多次复治组 PF（20.7±4.6）灌注值低于首次复治组（32.6±5.3），差异有统计学意义（P<0.05）；BF 值（25.8±3.2）略高于首次复治组（22.3±5.2），但差异无统计学意义。

本研究显示初治治愈组的整体灌注值（PF+BF）高于复治组，PF 值较高表明肺结核病灶高灌注状态与疗效有一定的关系，提示病灶局部肺循环血供丰富，血抗结核药血药浓度在此处比较高，病灶治愈的可能性大。复治组 PF 灌注值低，主要原因可能为炎症反应减少、消失或肉芽组织纤维化、血供减少，从而造成病灶内药物浓度低，细菌产生耐药，从而造成疗效差。多次复治组血管损伤更加严重，局部纤维化更加明显，形成了抗药壁垒。同时本研究的结果也表明，复治组病灶的 BF 值明显高于初治组，PI 值下降。BF 值升高者，表明支气管动脉（体循环）供血增多，可能是随着病灶进展，结核炎症病变产生的多种炎症因子，特别是血管内皮生长因子，在活动性肺结核患者的血液及病变组织中都有明显表达[11,12]，刺激支气管动脉与病灶相邻肺外体循环血管增生、扩张、通透性增加，病灶侵蚀肺动脉，甚至形成"支气管动脉—肺动脉瘘"，而体循环的压力明显大于肺循环，所以相对造成结核病灶中支气管动脉供血比例增加；但总体血液循环仍然较差，尤其是多次复治组的 BF 值亦高于首次复治组，提示病灶动态进展的变化，病理血管增多，此类患者用药效果往往不好。因此，肺动脉作为肺结核的主要滋养血管，其损伤程度决定了病灶能否达到有效的药物浓度，关乎整个肺结核化疗的疗效。支气管动脉在病灶发生的初始阶段虽能够提供少量供血，但随着病情进展，其病理血管有逐渐增多趋势，间接地反映了结核病灶的进展。

基于以上肺结核相关的 CT 灌注研究，表明 DI-CTP 可有效反映肺结核病灶血流动力学特征，可有效发现和定位结核伴发的体—肺动脉瘘，对肺结核大咯血患者的肺部血管异常做出评估，对指导下一步介入栓塞治疗有较大意义，并能定量反映出复治涂阳肺结核患者的血供特点，为肺结核疗效观察、预判提供了一种新的方法和思路。

参考文献

［1］　袁小东，敖国昆，全昌斌，等. 肺双重血供的 CT 灌注技术及其应用于肺结核的初步研究 ［J］. 中华临床医师杂志（电子版），2011，5（20）：5913 – 5918.

［2］　敖国昆，袁小东，全昌斌，等. 320 层肺双入口灌注技术对肺结核患者体循环动脉肺动脉瘘的诊断价值 ［J］. 2014 年结核病及肺部相关疾病影像学诊断与介入治疗高峰论坛资料汇编，126 – 129.

［3］　俞森洋. 呼吸危重病学 ［M］. 北京：中国协和医科大学出版社. 2008：156 – 158.

［4］　周辛姝. 肺结核咯血的发病机制及治疗 ［J］. 中国医药指南，2012，10（10）：463 – 464.

［5］　李慧，陈月芹，孙占国，等. MSCTA 在咯血诊疗中的应用价值 ［J］. 放射学实践，2012，27（4）：394 – 398.

［6］　宋美君，吴宏成，汤耀东，等. 多层螺旋支气管动脉造影与数字减影下经股动脉支气管动脉造影在

咯血诊治中的对比 [J]. 中国呼吸与危重监护杂志，2012，14（7）：378 – 381.

[7]　麻增林，张黎明. 多排螺旋对咯血患者肺部血管和实质的综合评价 [J]. 中华临床医师杂志（电子版），2011，5（1）：201 – 205.

[8]　姜静波，吴宏成，汤耀东，等. 支气管动脉造影与传统血管造影在咯血诊治中的对照研究 [J]. 实用现代医学，2013，25（1）：33 – 34.

[9]　中华人民共和国卫生部. 全国结核病耐药基线调查报告（2007 – 2008 年）[M]. 北京：人民卫生出版社，2010：24.

[10]　王黎霞. 中国耐多药结核病的控制亟待加强 [J]. 中华结核和呼吸杂志，2009，32（8）：561 – 563.

[11]　Alatas F，Aiatas O，Metintas M，et al. Vascular endothelial growthfactor levels in active pulmonary tuberculosis [J]. Chest，2004，125（6）：2156 – 2159.

[12]　沈兴华，陈兴年. 肺结核患者血清 VEGF 检测的临床分析 [J]. 临床肺科杂志，2010，15（9）：1322.

第四章

肺双重供血 CT 灌注技术临床病例展示

第一节　肺癌双重供血 CT 灌注病例

一、鳞癌

【病例 1】

患者，男。全身不适伴低热、咳嗽，偶伴咯血，3 个月，申请胸部 CT（图 4 - 1 - 1、图 4 - 1 - 2）。

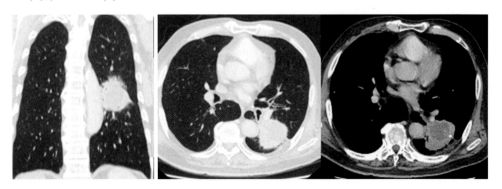

图 4 - 1 - 1　患者胸部 CT

CT 所见：左肺下叶背段可见大小约 5.6 cm×5.1 cm 软组织肿块影，边界毛糙，密度不均匀，中央部呈低密度区。其外侧可见点状钙化灶，邻近支气管截断。增强扫描病变外周明显强化，中央区未见明显强化

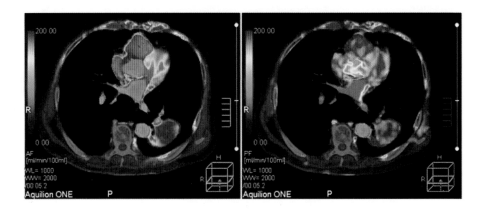

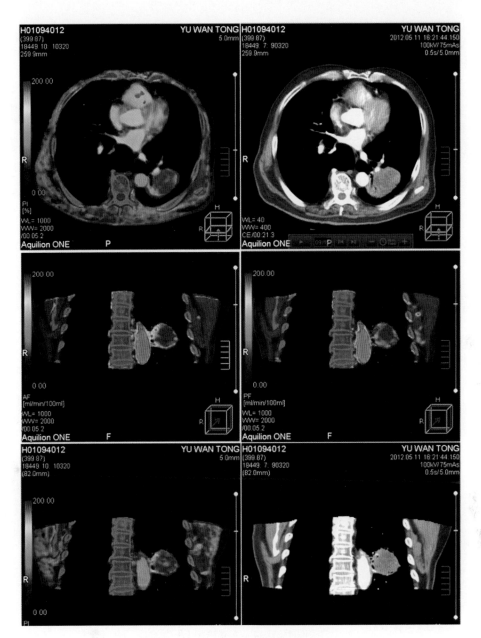

图 4 – 1 – 2　CT 灌注横断面及冠状面

病灶呈肺循环和体循环双重供血，以体循环（支气管动脉供血）占优势，中央坏死区无血供

术后病理所见参见图 4 – 1 – 3。

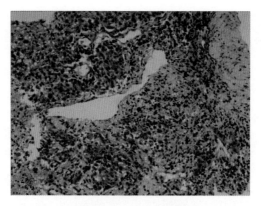

图 4 - 1 - 3 术后病理

肿瘤细胞呈片巢状排列，细胞异型性明显，可见
细胞间桥及坏死（HE×100）

最后诊断：低分化鳞癌。

【病例 2】

患者，男，73 岁。20d 前无明显诱因出现发热，体温最高达 38.5℃，无盗汗、寒战等
不适，伴咳嗽、咳痰，为草绿色黏痰，量不多，约 50 ml/d，与体位及时间无关，无胸痛、
痰中带血等不适。

申请胸部 CT（图 4 - 1 - 4 至图 4 - 1 - 6）。

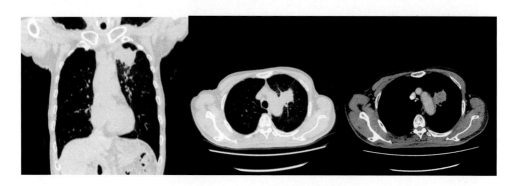

图 4 - 1 - 4 患者胸部 CT

左肺上叶纵隔旁可见一大小约 4.4 cm×3.7 cm 软组织密度影，其内密度不均，周围可见长毛刺影，相
应尖前段支气管闭塞。增强扫描病变呈明显不均匀强化

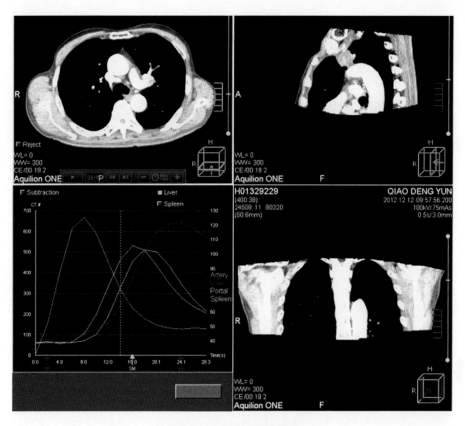

图 4 - 1 - 5　动态增强曲线

病灶强化曲线（红色）在体循环阶段上升斜率较大，说明其主要血供来源为支气管动脉

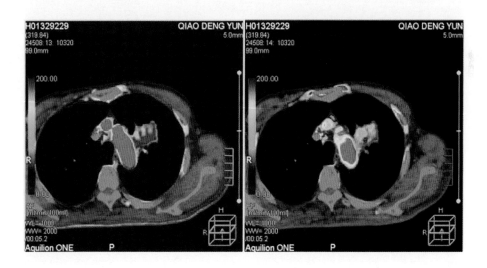

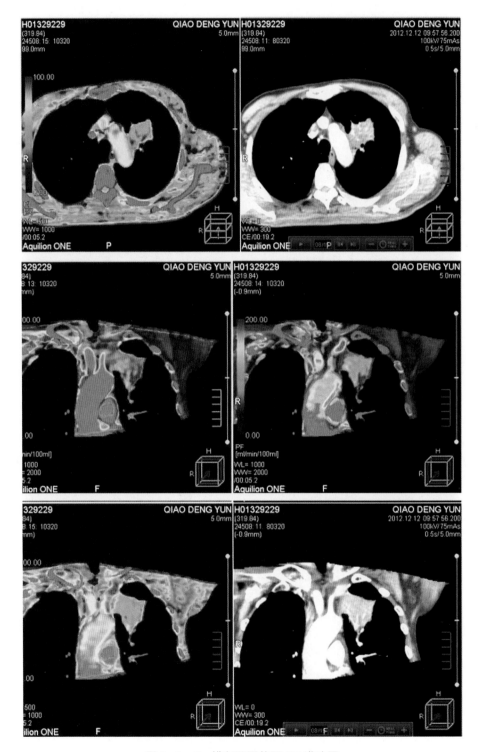

图 4 – 1 – 6　横断面冠状面 CT 灌注图

病灶肺动脉供血较少，支气管动脉供血很丰富术后病理所见参见图 4 - 1 - 7。

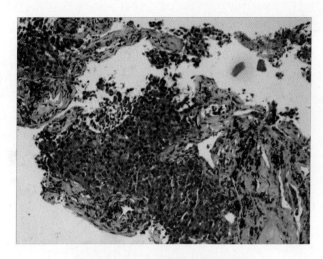

图 4 - 1 - 7　术后病理（HE × 100）

肿瘤细胞呈巢状排列，细胞异型性明显

诊断：中—高分化鳞癌。

【病例 3】

男，62 岁。右下肺中分化鳞癌，病灶大小 98.4 mm × 97.7 mm × 106.3 mm。CT 显示见图 4 - 1 - 8 至图 4 - 1 - 12。

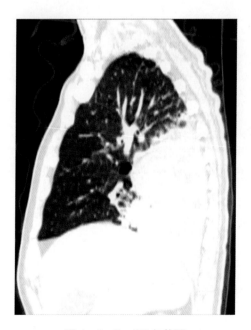

图 4 - 1 - 8　CT 矢状面

右肺下叶团片状病灶

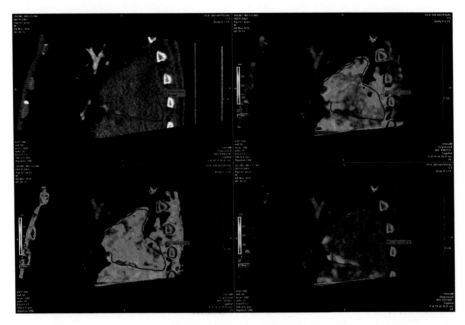

图4-1-9 矢状面灌注图

肺动脉血流量（pulmonary flow，PF）、支气管动脉血流量（bronchial flow，BF）、灌注指数（perfusion index，PI）分别为：68.1 ml/min/100 ml、115.7 ml/min/100 ml、36.4%

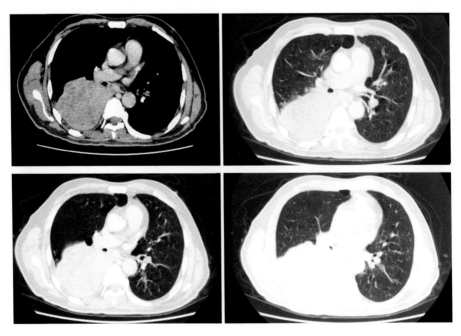

图4-1-10 CT横断面

右肺下叶团片状病灶，密度不均匀，边界尚清晰

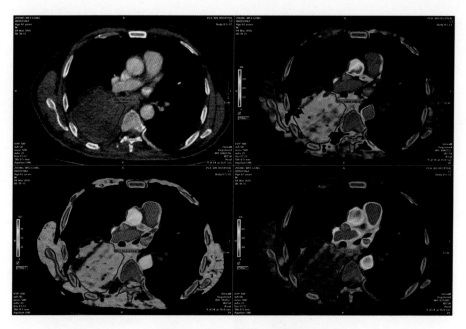

图 4 - 1 - 11 横断面灌注图

肺动脉血流量（pulmonary flow，PF）、支气管动脉血流量（bronchial flow，BF）、灌注指数
（perfusion index，PI）分别为：61.4 ml/min/100 ml、139.5 ml/min/100 ml、31.6%

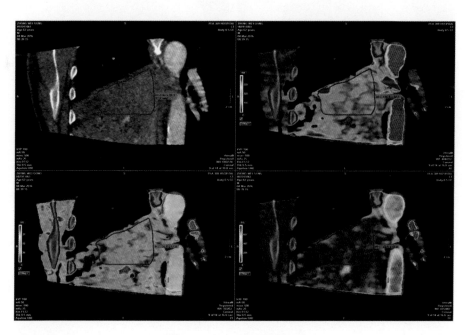

图 4 - 1 - 12 冠状面灌注图

肺动脉血流量（pulmonary flow，PF）、支气管动脉血流量（bronchial flow，BF）、灌注指数
（perfusion index，PI）分别为：62.5 ml/min/100 ml、135.5 ml/min/100 ml、31.9%

【病例4】

男，69岁，左上肺中分化鳞癌伴坏死，病灶大小 32.9 mm×37.9 mm×36.9 mm。CT 显示见图 4 -1 -13 至图 4 -1 -18。

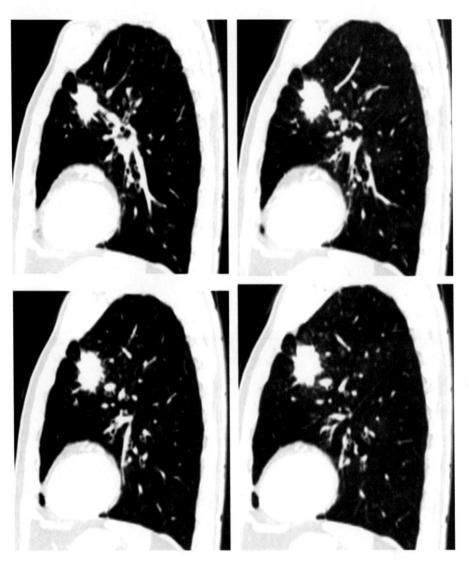

图4 -1 -13　CT 矢状面

左上肺分叶状肿块伴毛刺及胸膜凹陷征

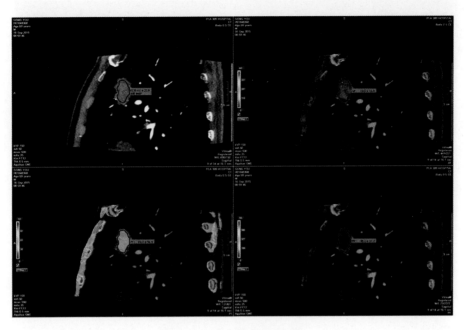

图 4 - 1 - 14 矢状面灌注图

肺动脉血流量（pulmonary flow，PF）、支气管动脉血流量（bronchial flow，BF）、灌注指数（perfusion index，PI）分别为：38.2 ml/min/100 ml、42.3 ml/min/100 ml、46.3%

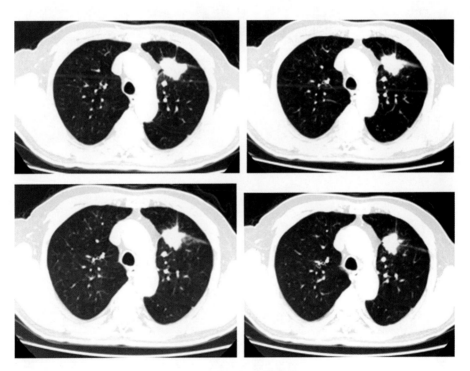

图 4 - 1 - 15 CT 横断面

左上肺分叶状肿块伴毛刺

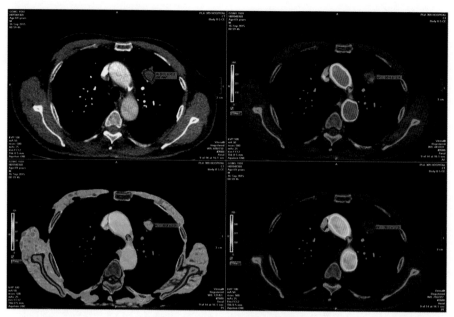

图 4-1-16 横断面灌注图

肺动脉血流量（pulmonary flow，PF）、支气管动脉血流量（bronchial flow，BF）、灌注指数（perfusion index，PI）分别为：36.2 ml/min/100 ml、55.4 ml/min/100 ml、39.0%

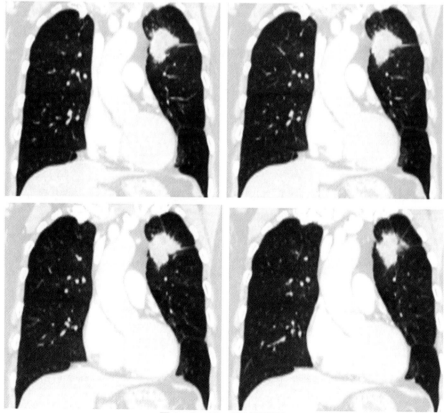

图 4-1-17 CT 冠状面

左上肺分叶状肿块伴毛刺

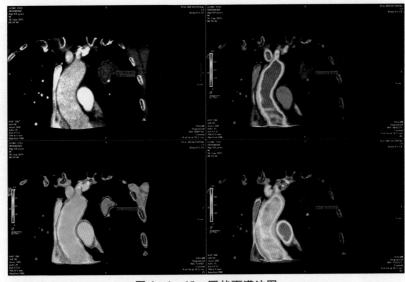

图 4 - 1 - 18 冠状面灌注图

肺动脉血流量（pulmonary flow，PF）、支气管动脉血流量（bronchial flow，BF）、灌注指数
（perfusion index，PI）分别为：33.7 ml/min/100 ml、45.6 ml/min/100 ml、42.8%

【病例5】

男，65 岁。右上低分化腺鳞癌坏死，51.6 mm×43.6 mm×42.8 mm。CT 显示见图 4 -
1 - 19 至图 4 - 1 - 24。

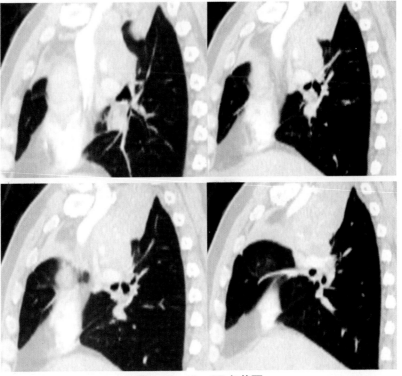

图 4 - 1 - 19 CT 矢状面

右上肺门旁肿块伴右上肺不张实变

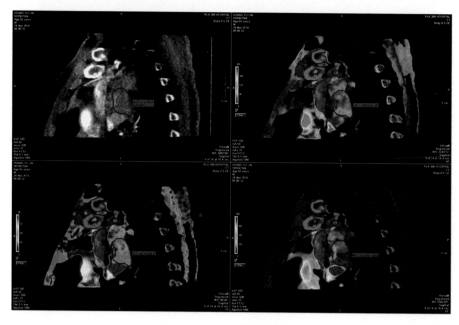

图 4 - 1 - 20　矢状面灌注图

肺动脉血流量（pulmonary flow，PF）、支气管动脉血流量（bronchial flow，BF）、灌注指数
（perfusion index，PI）分别为：74. 3ml/min/100 ml、55. 9 ml/min/100 ml、53. 8%

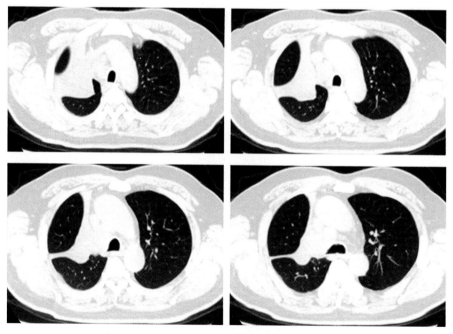

图 4 - 1 - 21　CT 横断面

右上肺门旁肿块伴右上肺不张实变

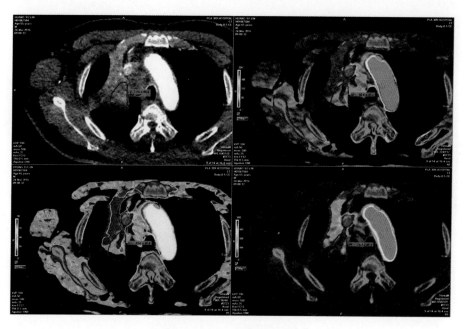

图 4 - 1 - 22　横断面灌注图

肺动脉血流量（pulmonary flow，PF）、支气管动脉血流量（bronchial flow，BF）、灌注指数（perfusion index，PI）分别为：110.8 ml/min/100 ml、46.4 ml/min/100 ml、61.7%

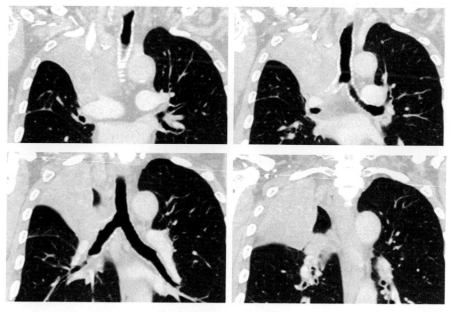

图 4 - 1 - 23　CT 冠状面

右上肺门旁肿块伴右上肺不张实变

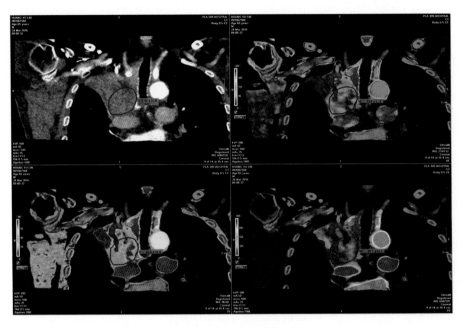

图 4 - 1 - 24　冠状面灌注图

肺动脉血流量（pulmonary flow，PF）、支气管动脉血流量（bronchial flow，BF）、灌注指数（perfusion index，PI）分别为：81.2 ml/min/100 ml、45.9 ml/min/100 ml、60.6%

二、腺癌

【病例 1】

男，64 岁。9 个月前无明显诱因左侧胸痛就诊，病理诊断为低分化腺癌。CT 显示见图 4 - 1 - 25 至图 4 - 1 - 27。

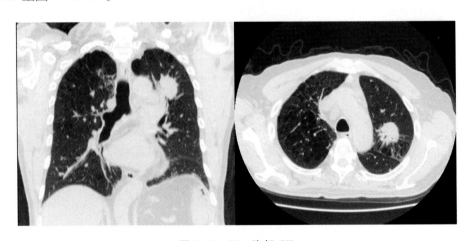

图 4 - 1 - 25　胸部 CT

左肺上叶可见一类圆形高密度影，边界可见多发细小毛刺影，内密度尚均匀

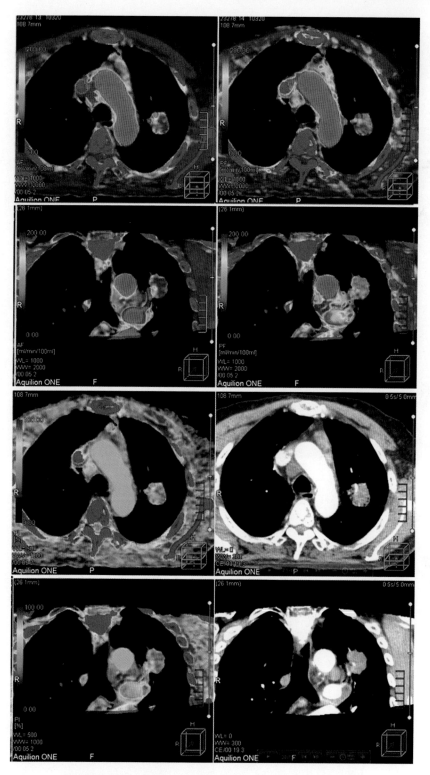

图 4 – 1 – 26　横断面 CT 灌注（CT Perfusion，CTp）图

病变以支气管动脉供血占绝对优势，边缘可见少许肺动脉供血

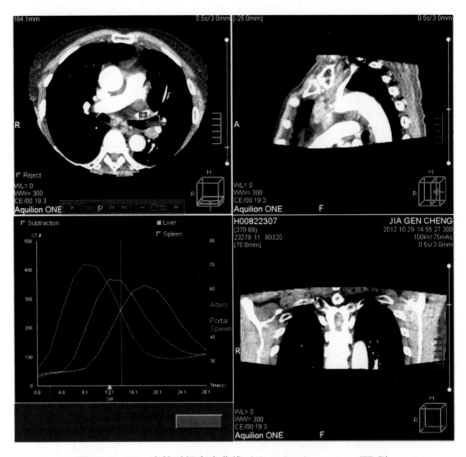

图4-1-27 病灶时间密度曲线（time density curve，TDC）

体循环阶段病灶曲线（红色）上升的斜率略大，提示体动脉（支气管动脉）血供略高于肺动脉血供

术后病理见图4-1-28。

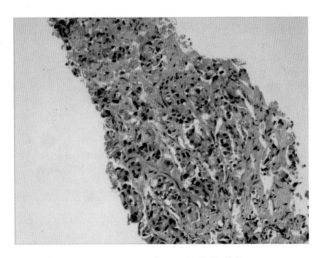

图4-1-28 病理：低分化腺癌

【病例2】

男，52 岁。咳嗽、咯血、胸闷不适 2 年余。CT 显示见图 4−1−29 至图 4−1−32。

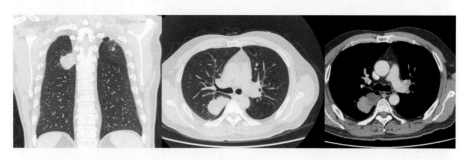

图 4−1−29　CT

右肺上叶后段斜裂旁可见团块状软组织密度影，内密度不均，内侧密度较低，增强扫描未见
明显强化，外侧部分明显强化，病变呈分叶性生长

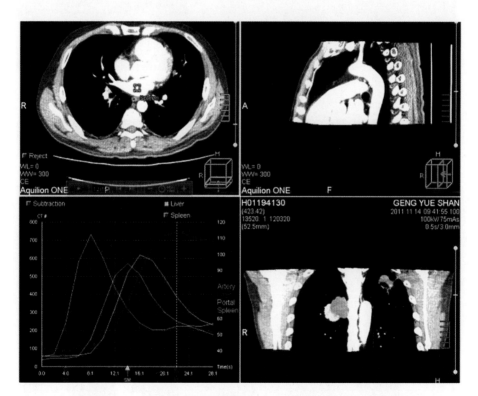

图 4−1−30　病灶时间密度曲线（Time density curve，TDC）

体循环阶段病灶曲线（红色）上升的斜率明显大于肺循环阶段，提示体动脉（支气管动脉）血
供高于肺动脉血供

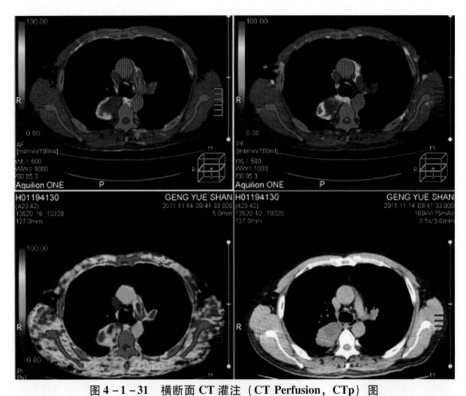

图 4 – 1 – 31 横断面 CT 灌注 (CT Perfusion, CTp) 图

病变内侧部分 (结核) 未见明显血供, 外侧部分 (腺癌) 以支气管动脉供血占明显优势

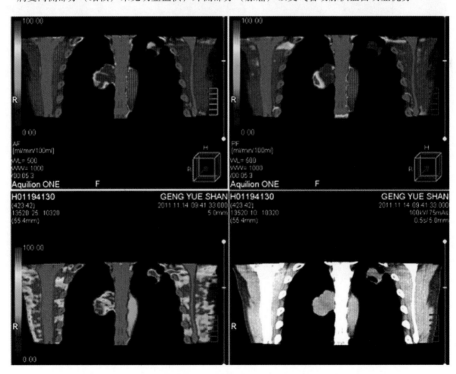

图 4 – 1 – 32 冠状面 CT 灌注 (CT Perfusion, CTp) 图

病灶上内侧部分 (结核) 未见明显血供, 下外侧部分 (腺癌) 以支气管动脉供血占明显优势

【病例 3】

女，63 岁。咳嗽、偶有痰中带血，乏力，食欲不振 2 个月余。CT 显示参见图 4 - 1 - 33 至图 4 - 1 - 35。

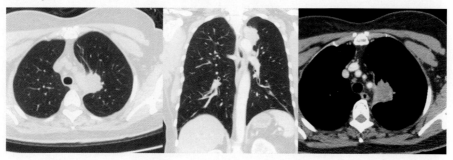

图 4 - 1 - 33　胸部 CT

左肺上叶纵隔旁可见不规则软组织影，直径约 3.4 cm，周边可见分叶、毛刺影，增强可见局部明显强化

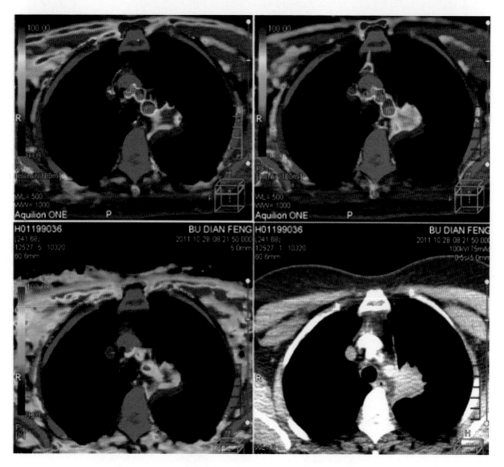

图 4 - 1 - 34　横断面 CT 灌注（CT Perfusion，CTp）图

病灶支气管动脉供血占明显优势

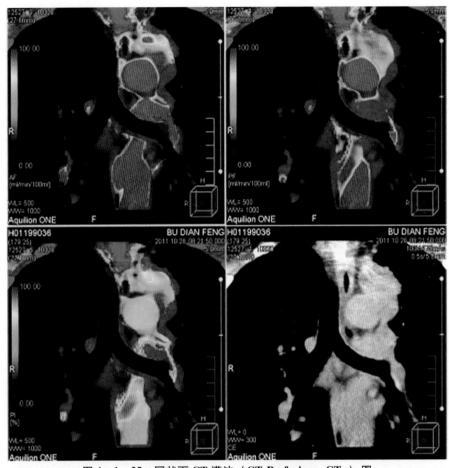

图 4 - 1 - 35　冠状面 CT 灌注（CT Perfusion，CTp）图

病变以支气管动脉供血占主要优势，肺动脉供血期边缘可见少许血供

术后病理见图 4 - 1 - 36。

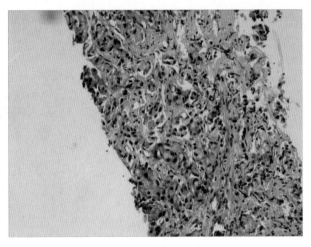

图 4 - 1 - 36　术后病理（HE × 100）

肿瘤细胞呈片巢状，细胞异型性明显，可见坏死及角化

诊断：中分化腺癌。

【病例 4】

女，44 岁。左上肺中—低分化腺癌，病灶大小为 32.1 mm×30.6 mm×28.4 mm。CT 显示参见图 4-1-37 至图 4-1-42。

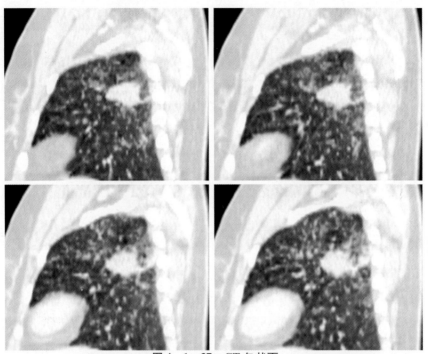

图 4-1-37　CT 矢状面

左上肺不规则形病灶，边界清

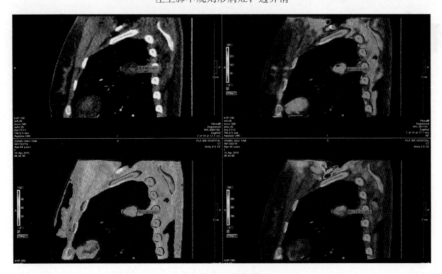

图 4-1-38　矢状面灌注图

肺动脉血流量（pulmonary flow，PF）、支气管动脉血流量（bronchial flow，BF）、灌注指数（perfusion index，PI）分别为：151.5 ml/min/100 ml、164.1 ml/min/100 ml、48.6%

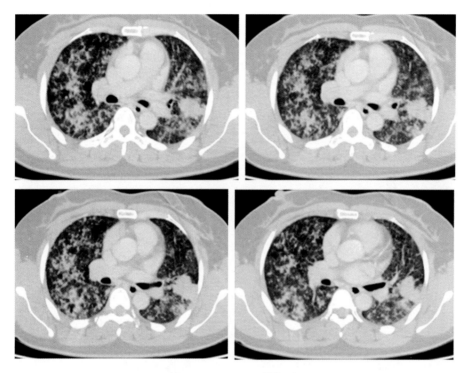

图 4 - 1 - 39　CT 横断面

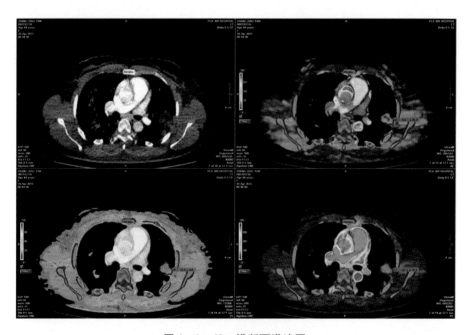

图 4 - 1 - 40　横断面灌注图

　　肺动脉血流量（pulmonary flow，PF）、支气管动脉血流量（bronchial flow，BF）、灌注指数（perfusion index，PI）分别为：121.6 ml/min/100 ml、136.9 ml/min/100 ml、46.7%

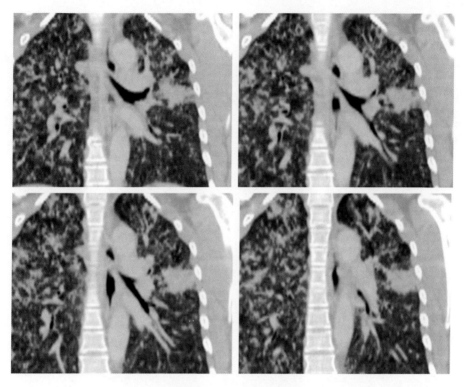

图 4 - 1 - 41 CT 冠状面

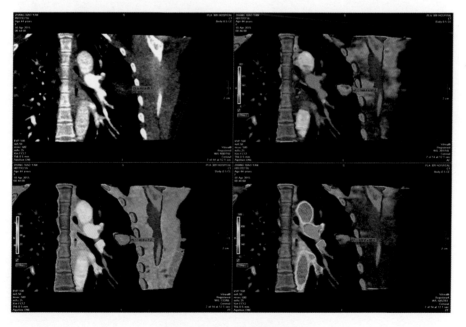

图 4 - 1 - 42 冠状面灌注图

肺动脉血流量（pulmonary flow，PF）、支气管动脉血流量（bronchial flow，BF）、灌注指数（perfusion index，PI）分别为：127.6 ml/min/100 ml、146.4 ml/min/100 ml、45.8%

【病例 5】

女，77 岁。右上肺中一高分化腺癌，病灶大小为 27.4 mm×33.3 mm×35.4 mm。CT 显示参见图 4-1-43 至图 4-1-48。

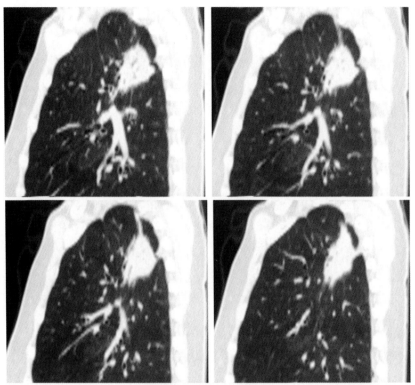

图 4-1-43　CT 矢状面

右上肺团片状病灶伴胸膜凹陷

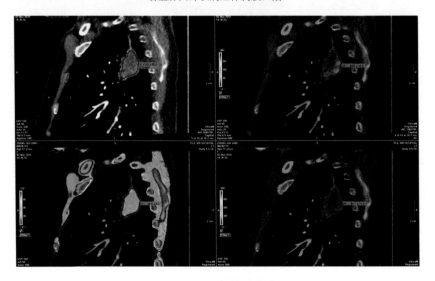

图 4-1-44　矢状面灌注图

肺动脉血流量（pulmonary flow，PF）、支气管动脉血流量（bronchial flow，BF）、灌注指数（perfusion index，PI）分别为：40.4 ml/min/100 ml、40.9 ml/min/100 ml、51.1%

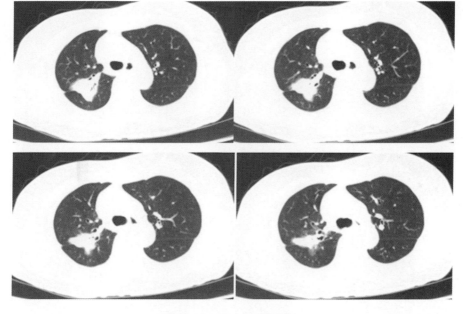

图 4 - 1 - 45　CT 横断面

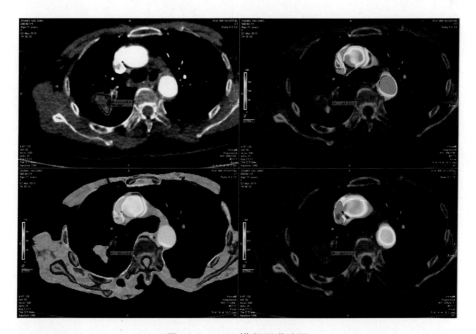

图 4 - 1 - 46　横断面灌注图

肺动脉血流量（pulmonary flow，PF）、支气管动脉血流量（bronchial flow，BF）、灌注指数（perfusion index，PI）分别为：31.1 ml/min/100 ml、38.0 ml/min/100 ml、45.0%

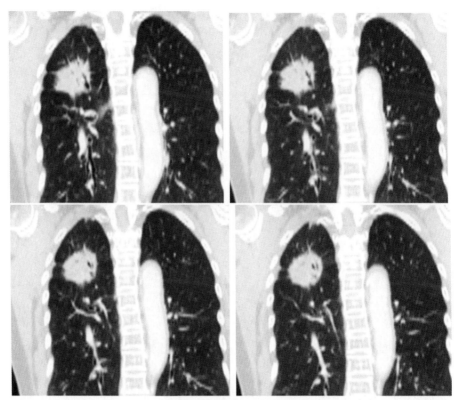

图 4 - 1 - 47　CT 冠状面

右上肺肿块伴胸膜凹陷

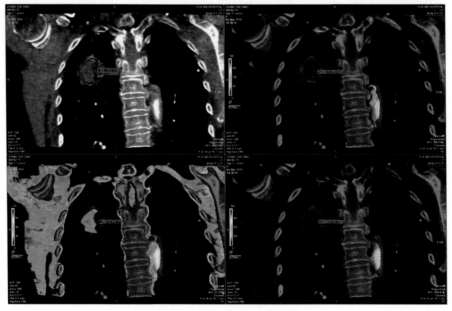

图 4 - 1 - 48　横断面灌注图

肺动脉血流量（pulmonary flow，PF）、支气管动脉血流量（bronchial flow，BF）、灌注指数（perfusion index，PI）分别为：22.0 ml/min/100 ml、29.6 ml/min/100 ml、42.5%

三、小细胞肺癌

【病例1】

患者，男，47岁。无明显诱因出现刺激性干咳2个月，偶有白黏痰，无痰中带血，无胸闷、憋气，无低热、盗汗，自行抗感染、止咳治疗效果不佳。病理诊断为左下肺小细胞癌。CT显示见图4-1-49至图4-1-51。

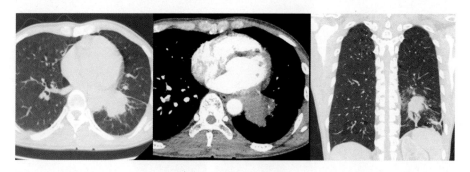

图4-1-49　胸部CT

左肺下叶可见不规则软组织影，大小约4.7 cm×4.2 cm×6.9 cm，周边可见分叶，病变包绕肺静脉，并向纵隔内生长；左肺下叶支气管部分闭塞。增强扫描呈明显强化

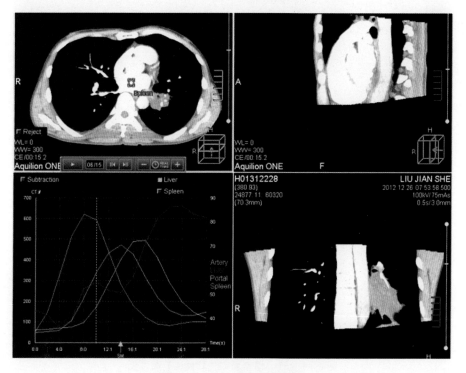

图4-1-50　动态增强曲线

病灶TDC呈双斜坡状上升，提示病灶接受肺动脉和支气管动脉的双重供血

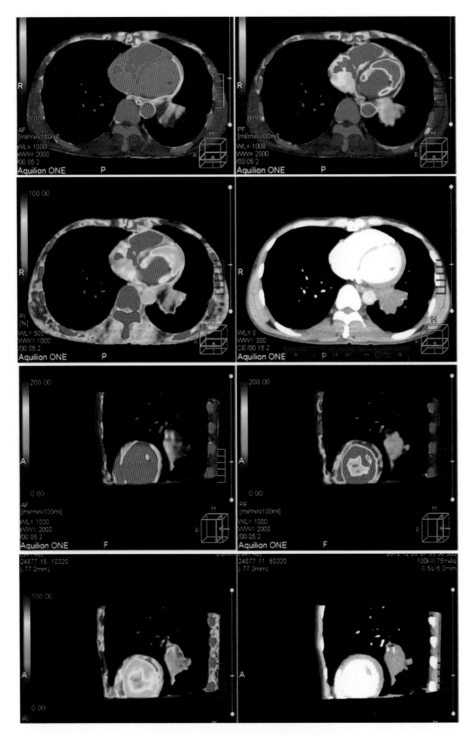

图4-1-51 横断面和矢状面CT灌注图

支气管动脉供血（体循环）占绝对优势

【病例 2】

男，46 岁。左肺尖小细胞癌。CT 显示见图 4 – 1 – 52 至图 4 – 1 – 53。

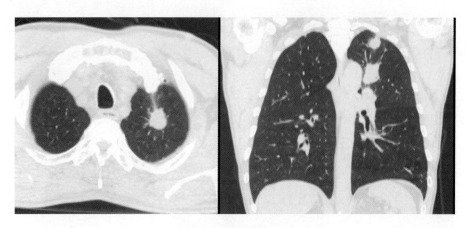

图 4 – 1 – 52　胸部 CT

左肺上肺可见两个大小不等类圆形软组织密度影，伴毛刺，部分与胸膜形成牵拉。增强扫描病变明显强化

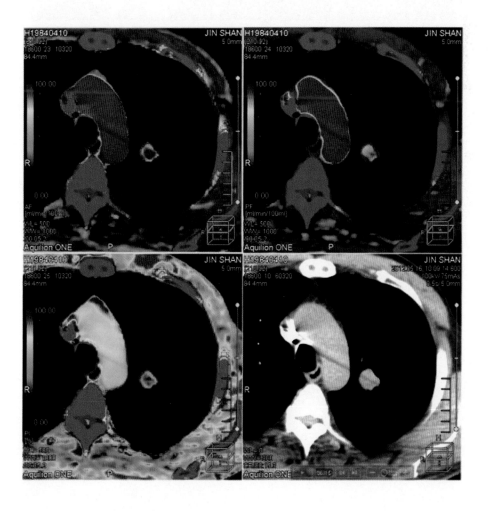

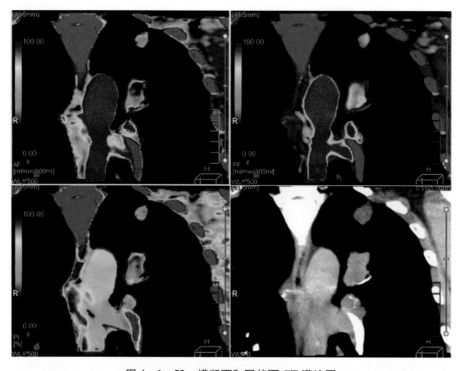

图 4 - 1 - 53　横断面和冠状面 CT 灌注图

两处病灶血供丰富，为肺动脉及支气管动脉双重供血，均以支气管动脉血供略占优势

【病例 3】

男，75 岁。左下肺小细胞肺癌，病灶大小为 53.1 mm × 51.2 mm × 45.5 mm。CT 显示见图 4 - 1 - 54 至图 4 - 1 - 59。

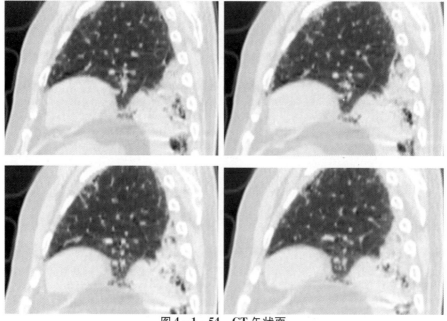

图 4 - 1 - 54　CT 矢状面

左肺下叶基底段肿块

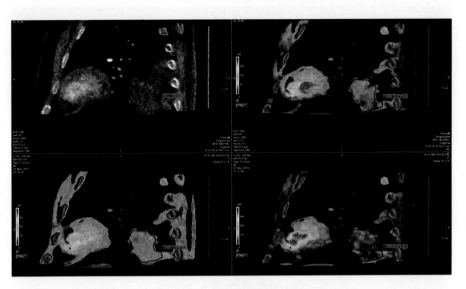

图 4 - 1 - 55　矢状面灌注图

肺动脉血流量（pulmonary flow，PF）、支气管动脉血流量（bronchial flow，BF）、灌注指数（perfusion index，PI）分别为：85.5 ml/min/100 ml、81.5 ml/min/100 ml、51.2%

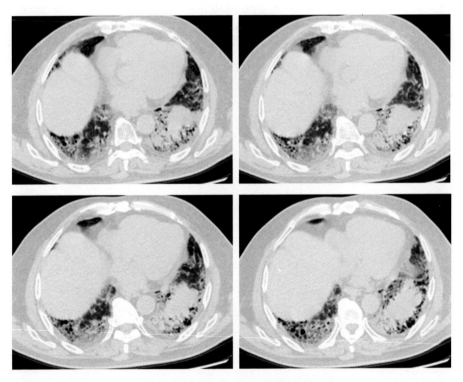

图 4 - 1 - 56　CT 横断面

左下肺基底段肿块

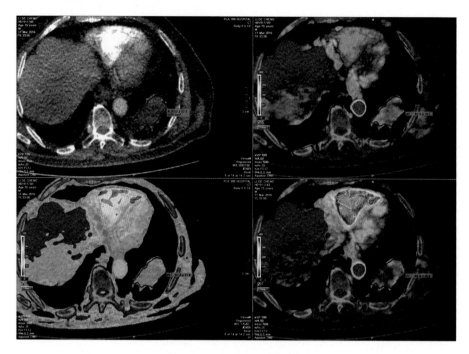

图4-1-57 横断面灌注图

肺动脉血流量（pulmonary flow，PF）、支气管动脉血流量（bronchial flow，BF）、灌注指数（perfusion index，PI）分别为：77.3 ml/min/100 ml、94.6 ml/min/100 ml、46.0%

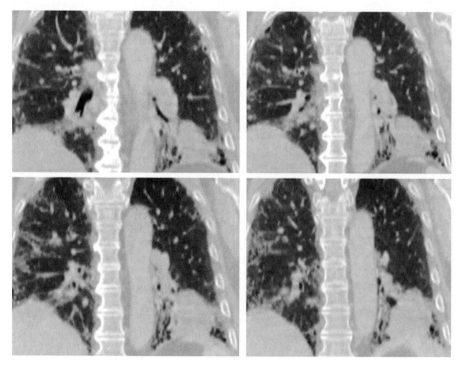

图4-1-58 CT冠状面

肿块位于左侧膈面上方

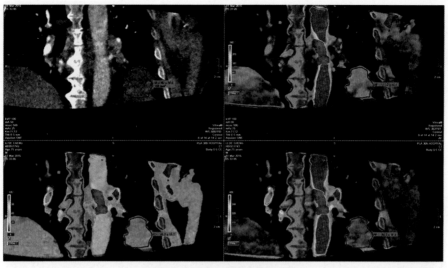

图 4 - 1 - 59　冠状面灌注图

肺动脉血流量（pulmonary flow，PF）、支气管动脉血流量（bronchial flow，BF）、灌注指数（perfusion index，PI）分别为：86.2 ml/min/100 ml、111.2 ml/min/100 ml、45.3%

【病例 4】

女，63 岁。右下小细胞肺癌，病灶大小为 44.8 mm×56 mm×48.7 mm。CT 显示见图 4 - 1 - 60 至图 4 - 1 - 65。

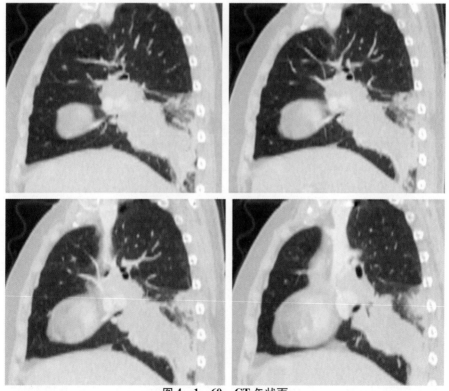

图 4 - 1 - 60　CT 矢状面

右肺下叶背段肿块

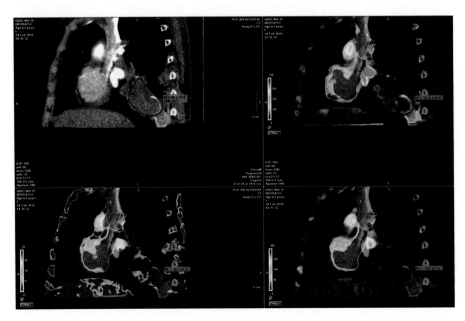

图 4 – 1 – 61　矢状面灌注图

肺动脉血流量（pulmonary flow，PF）、支气管动脉血流量（bronchial flow，BF）、灌注指数（perfusion index，PI）分别为：9.4 ml/min/100 ml、86.9 ml/min/100 ml、9.1%

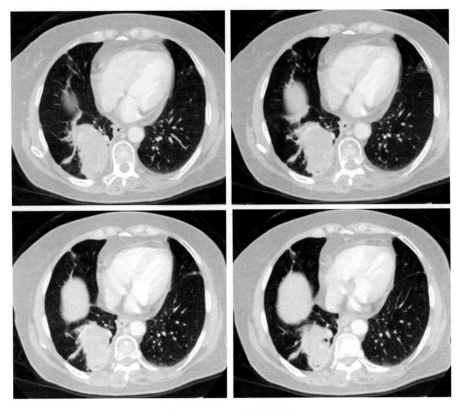

图 4 – 1 – 62　CT 横断面

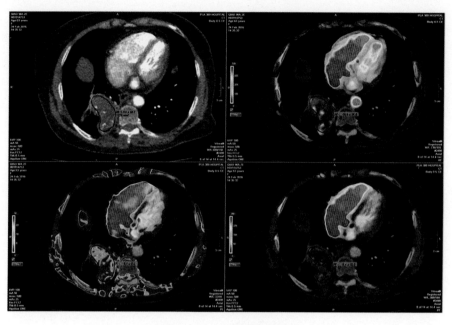

图 4 - 1 - 63　横断面灌注图

肺动脉血流量（pulmonary flow，PF）、支气管动脉血流量（bronchial flow，BF）、灌注指数
（perfusion index，PI）分别为：3.7 ml/min/100 ml、72.8 ml/min/100 ml、4.7%

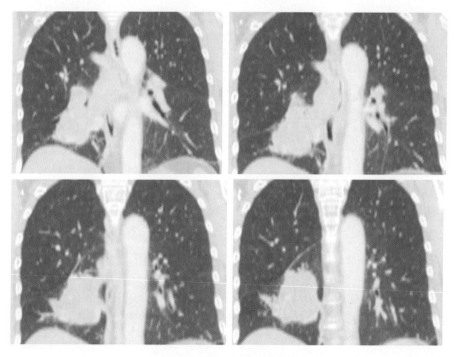

图 4 - 1 - 64　CT 冠状面

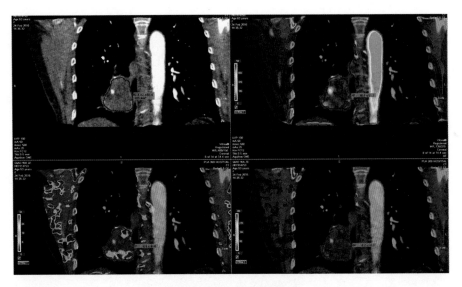

图 4 – 1 – 65　冠状面灌注图

肺动脉血流量（pulmonary flow，PF）、支气管动脉血流量（bronchial flow，BF）、灌注指数
（perfusion index，PI）分别为：6.4 ml/min/100 ml、88.6 ml/min/100 ml、6.9%

【病例 5】

女，66 岁。左上小细胞肺癌，病灶大小为 81.9 mm×78.3 mm×83.6 mm。CT 显示见图
4 – 1 – 66 至图 4 – 1 – 70。

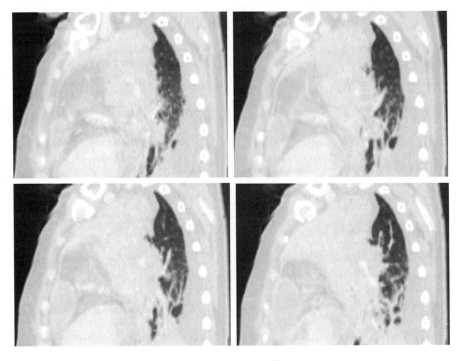

图 4 – 1 – 66　CT 矢状面

左肺上叶肺门旁肿块伴左上肺不张实变

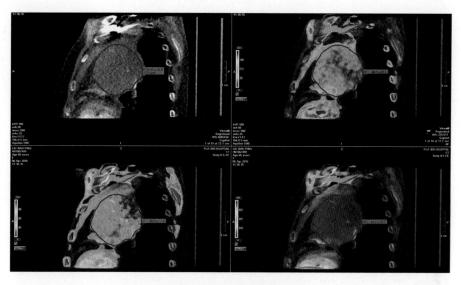

图 4 - 1 - 67　矢状面灌注图

肺动脉血流量（pulmonary flow，PF）、支气管动脉血流量（bronchial flow，BF）、灌注指数（perfusion index，PI）分别为：47.6 ml/min/100 ml、51.2 ml/min/100 ml、46.8%

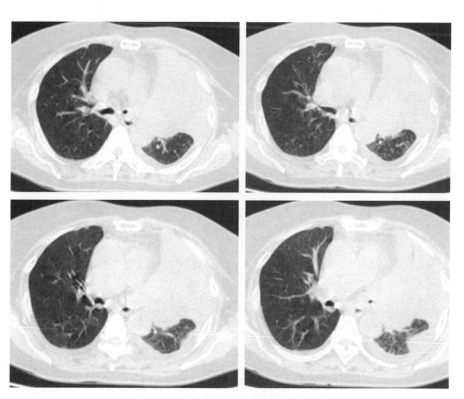

图 4 - 1 - 68　CT 横断面

左肺门占位伴左上肺实变

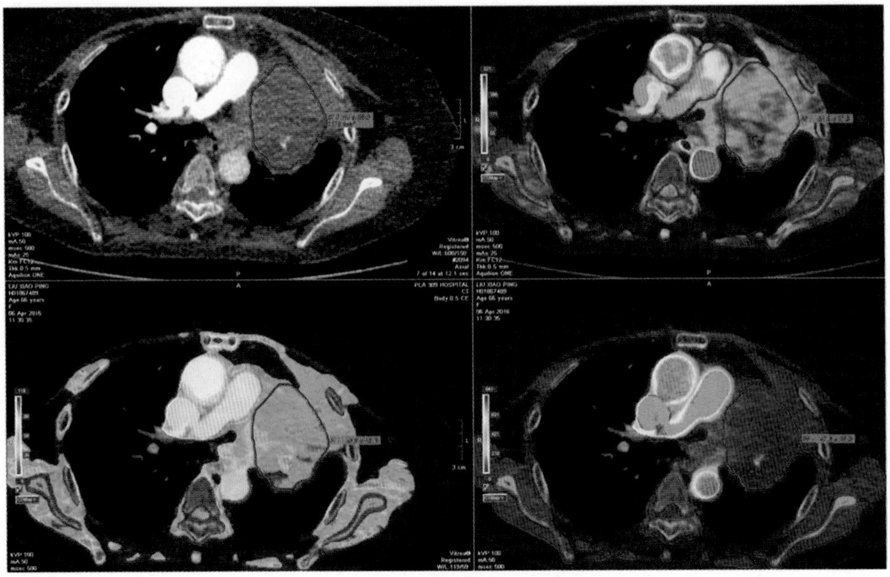

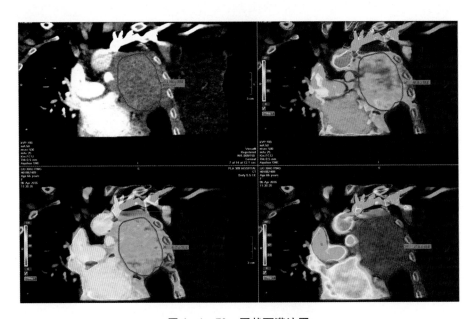

图 4 - 1 - 69　横断面灌注图

肺动脉血流量（pulmonary flow，PF）、支气管动脉血流量（bronchial flow，BF）、灌注指数
（perfusion index，PI）分别为：40.7 ml/min/100 ml、63.0 ml/min/100 ml、39.7%

图 4 - 1 - 70　冠状面灌注图

肺动脉血流量（pulmonary flow，PF）、支气管动脉血流量（bronchial flow，BF）、灌注指数
（perfusion index，PI）分别为：47.6 ml/min/100 ml、69.6 ml/min/100 ml、41.7%

四、转移瘤

【病例 1】

患者，男，22 岁。肝肿瘤切除术后 3 年，肝肿瘤介入治疗术后 1 个月余，左肺下叶转移瘤。CT 显示见图 4 – 1 – 71 至图 4 – 1 – 72。

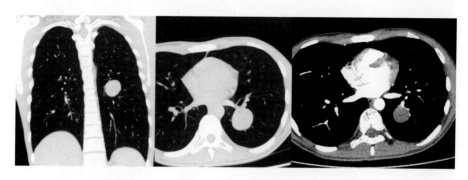

图 4 – 1 – 71　胸部 CT

左肺下叶背段可见一类圆形软组织肿块影，边界光滑，大小约 3.1 cm×2.6 cm，内密度均匀，CT 值约 47 cm，呈明显强化

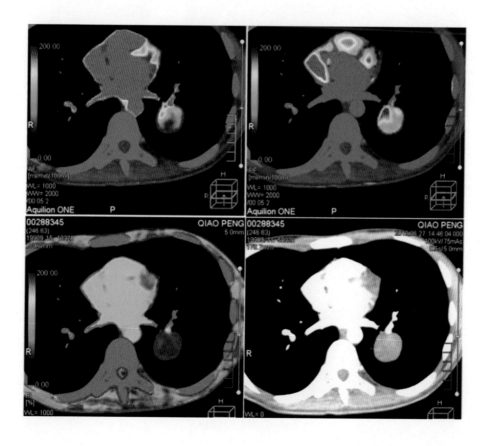

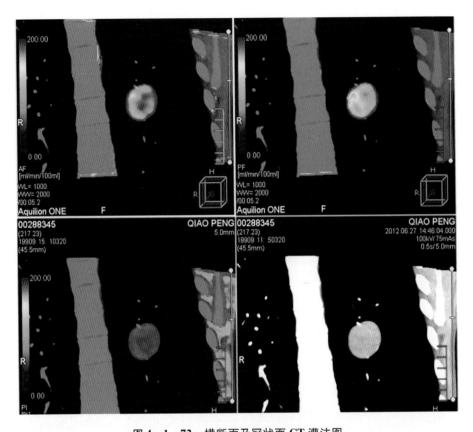

图 4 - 1 - 72 横断面及冠状面 CT 灌注图

病变血供丰富，肺动脉及支气管动脉期均有供血，以支气管动脉期供血占优势

【病例2】

患者，男，58岁。患者于2012年4月无明显诱因出现头晕、头痛不适症状，就诊查头颅 CT 提示头颅转移瘤可能性大，立即住院治疗。右肺病灶手术病理：转移瘤。CT 显示见图 4 - 1 - 73 至图 4 - 1 - 74。

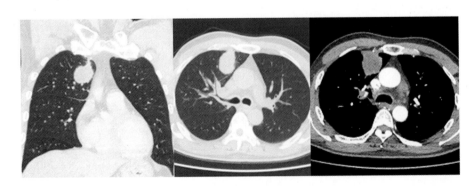

图 4 - 1 - 73 胸部 CT

右肺上叶前段见不规则软组织肿块影，呈浅分叶，伴毛刺，大小约为 3.2 cm×4.4 cm

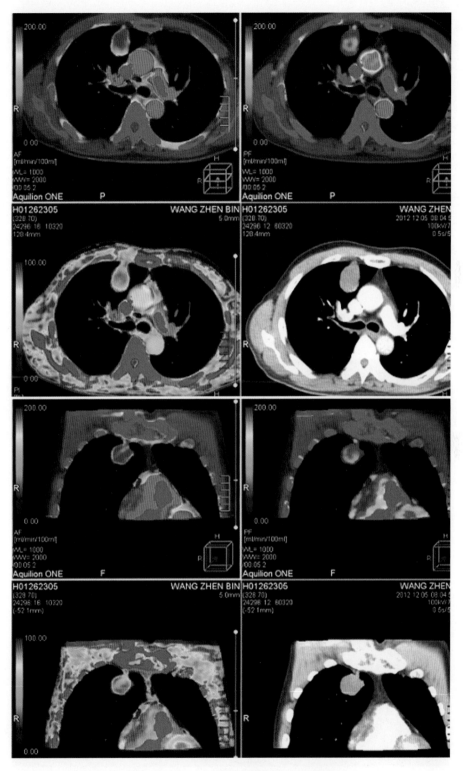

图 4 - 1 - 74　CT 灌注横断面及冠状面图

病灶以支气管动脉供血占主要优势，病灶边缘见少量肺动脉供血

【病例 3】

患者，男，60 岁。右肺下叶转移瘤。CT 显示见图 4 – 1 – 75 至图 4 – 1 – 76。

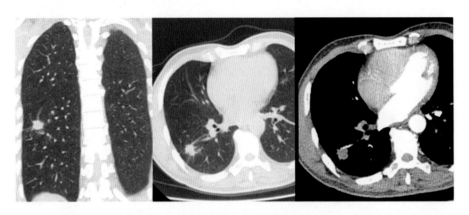

图 4 – 1 – 75　胸部 CT

右肺下叶背段邻近胸膜下结节灶，大小约 1.65 cm × 1.75 cm，可见毛刺及分叶，增强可见轻度强化

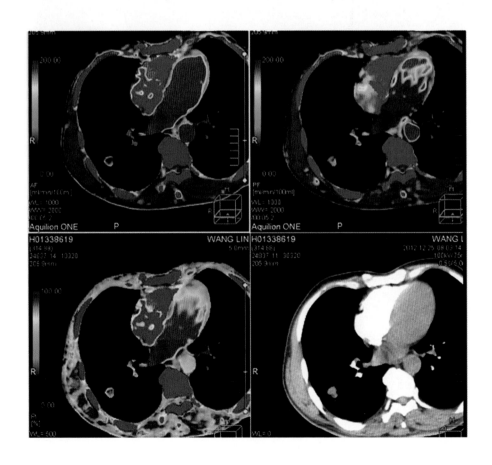

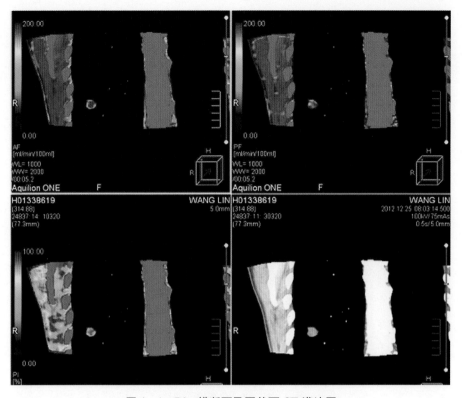

图4-1-76 横断面及冠状面CT灌注图

病变周边可见少许肺动脉供血，中央部分为支气管动脉供血占优势

五、神经内分泌癌

患者，男，51岁。无明显诱因咳嗽、咳痰1年，无胸痛、咯血，无发热、盗汗，无腹痛、腹泻，无关节及肌肉酸痛。自服抗炎、止咳药物后，病情好转，半个月前无明显诱因症状加重；手术病理为神经内分泌癌。CT显示见图4-1-77至图4-1-79。

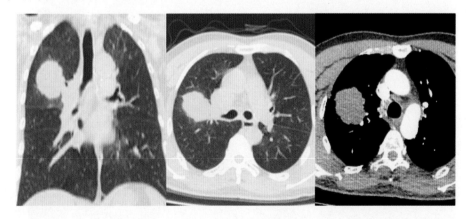

图4-1-77 胸部CT

右肺上叶可见不规则软组织影，其内密度均匀，最大径约4.7 cm×6.1 cm×4.9 cm，周边可见小毛刺，增强可见不均匀强化，右上叶支气管远端狭窄

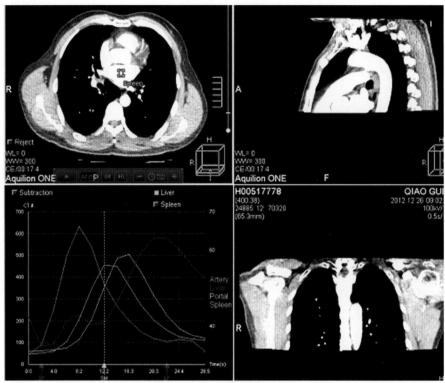

图 4 - 1 - 78   动态增强曲线

病灶 TDC 呈双斜坡状上升，以体循环阶段斜率较大，提示病灶接受肺循环和体循环双重供血，以体循环供血为主

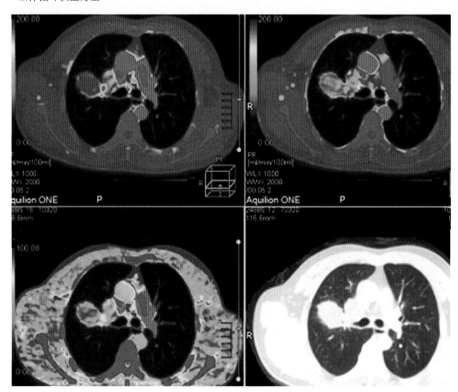

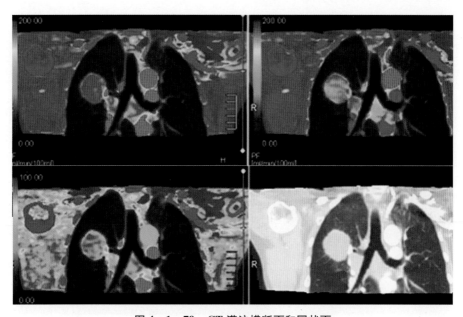

图 4 - 1 - 79　CT 灌注横断面和冠状面

病变以支气管动脉供血占优势，肺动脉血供较弱

六、淋巴瘤

男，27 岁。右肺上叶前段淋巴瘤，病灶大小为 82.6 mm×62.1 mm×76.1 mm。CT 显示见图 4 - 1 - 80 至图 4 - 1 - 85。

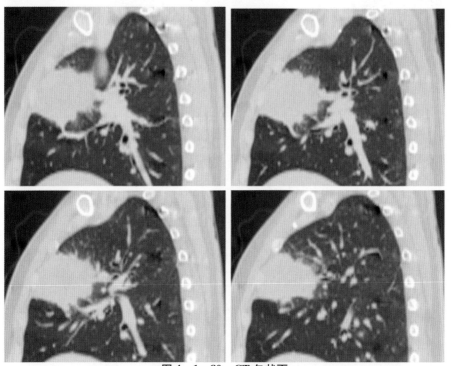

图 4 - 1 - 80　CT 矢状面

右肺上叶前段团片状病灶，边界清

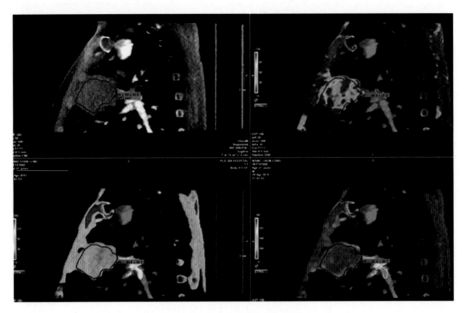

图 4 - 1 - 81　冠状面灌注图

肺动脉血流量（pulmonary flow，PF）、支气管动脉血流量（bronchial flow，BF）、灌注指数
（perfusion index，PI）分别为：86.2 ml/min/100 ml、48.9 ml/min/100 ml、67.6%

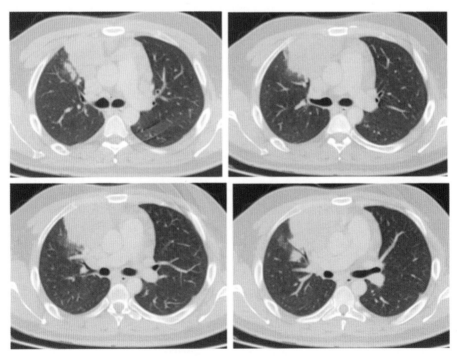

图 4 - 1 - 82　CT 横断面

右肺上叶前段病灶

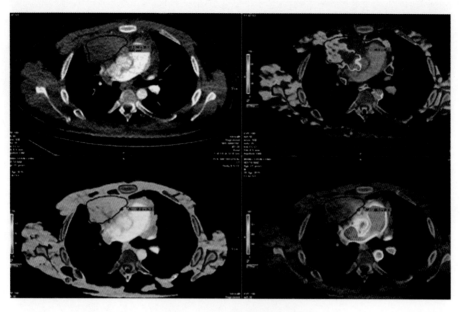

图 4 - 1 - 83　横断面灌注图

肺动脉血流量（pulmonary flow，PF）、支气管动脉血流量（bronchial flow，BF）、灌注指数
（perfusion index，PI）分别为：91.5 ml/min/100 ml、66.3 ml/min/100 ml、61.9%

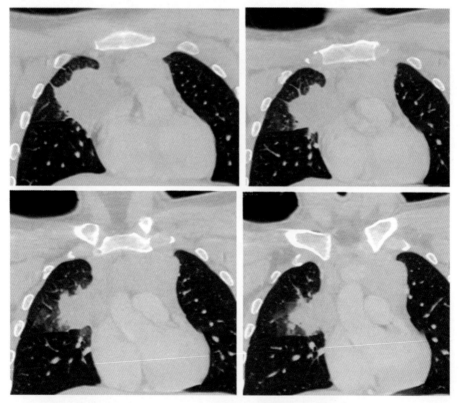

图 4 - 1 - 84　CT 冠状面

右肺上叶前段肿块，病灶位于水平裂上方，呈分叶状

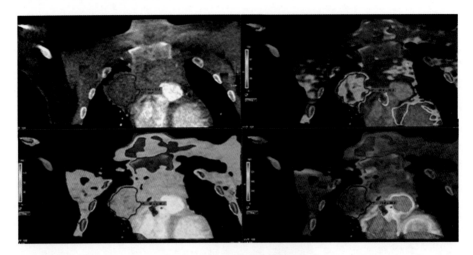

图 4 - 1 - 85　冠状面灌注图

肺动脉血流量（pulmonary flow，PF）、支气管动脉血流量（bronchial flow，BF）、灌注指数（perfusion index，PI）分别为：91.5 ml/min/100 ml、66.3 ml/min/100 ml、61.9%

七、硬化性肺泡细胞瘤

女，44 岁。左肺上叶硬化性肺泡细胞瘤，病灶大小约为 67.3 mm × 62 mm × 66.8 mm。CT 显示见图 4 - 1 - 86 至图 4 - 1 - 91。

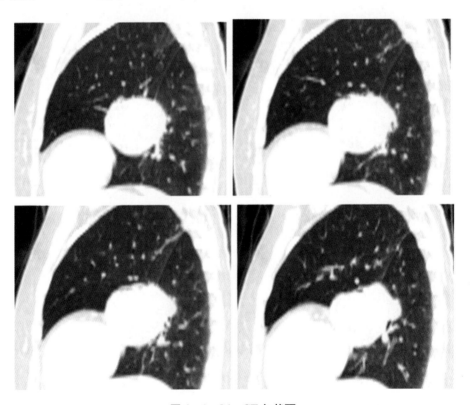

图 4 - 1 - 86　CT 矢状面

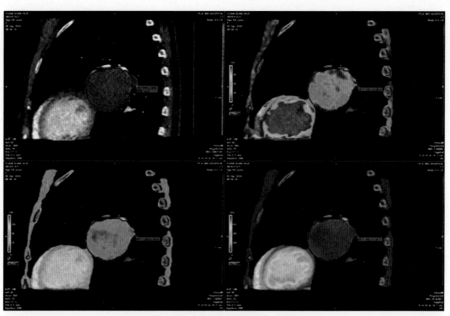

图 4 - 1 - 87　矢状面灌注图

肺动脉血流量（pulmonary flow，PF）、支气管动脉血流量（bronchial flow，BF）、灌注指数（perfusion index，PI）分别为：59. 7 ml/min/100 ml、77. 6 ml/min/100 ml、40. 2%

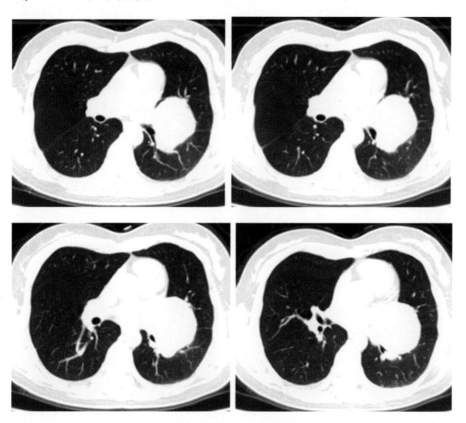

图 4 - 1 - 88　CT 横断面

肿瘤呈类圆形，边界清晰光整

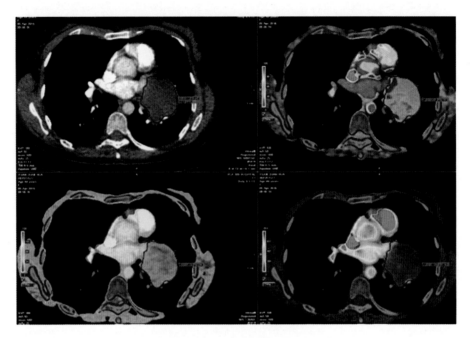

图 4 - 1 - 89 横断面灌注图

肺动脉血流量（pulmonary flow，PF）、支气管动脉血流量（bronchial flow，BF）、灌注指数
（perfusion index，PI）分别为：62.2 ml/min/100 ml、73.1 ml/min/100 ml、45.0%

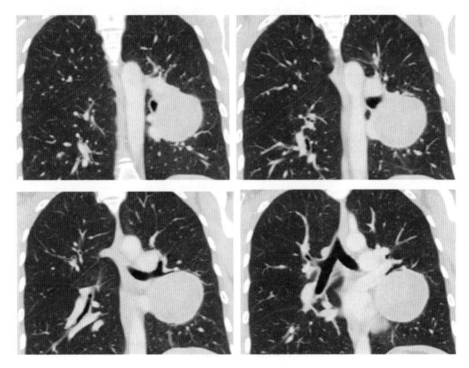

图 4 - 1 - 90 CT 冠状面

肿块位于左肺上叶舌段

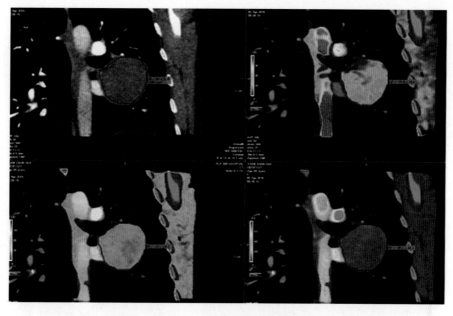

图4-1-91　横断面灌注图

肺动脉血流量（pulmonary flow，PF）、支气管动脉血流量（bronchial flow，BF）、灌注指数（perfusion index，PI）分别为：60.4 ml/min/100 ml、77.8 ml/min/100 ml、43.4%

第二节　肺结核的双重供血CT灌注

一、肺内结核病灶

【病例1】

男性，32岁。临床确诊为肺结核1年。CT显示见图4-2-1至图4-2-2。

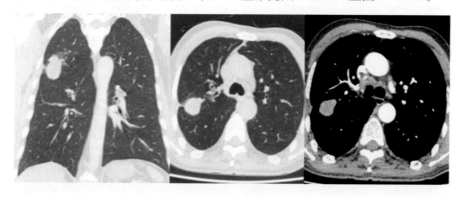

图4-2-1　胸部CT

右肺上叶后段近斜裂胸膜可见不规则混渃密度影，大小约6.5 cm×2.5 cm，局部可见钙化灶及小空泡征，周边可见胸膜牵拉征象，邻近支气管局部轻度扩张。增强未见明显强化

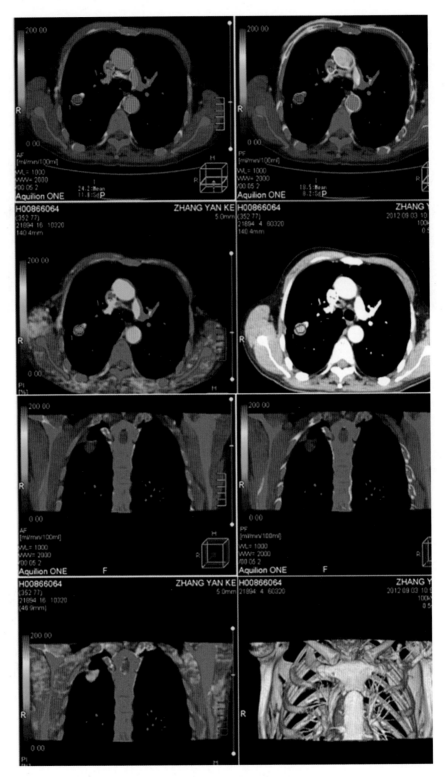

图 4 - 2 - 2　CT 灌注横断面及冠状面

病变为乏血供，两个循环均未见明显血供，肺循环略占优势

【病例2】

患者，女64岁。胸闷、乏力、低热入院，申请胸部CT。CT显示见图4-2-3至图4-2-4。

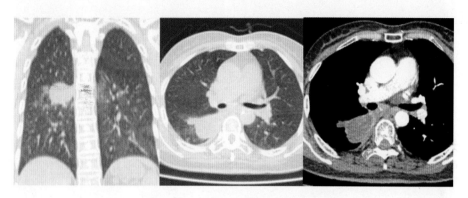

图4-2-3　CT扫描

右肺下叶背段可见一大小约3.1 cm×3.0 cm软组织密度灶，边界较清，内密度均匀，相应背段支气管变窄。增强扫描呈轻度强化

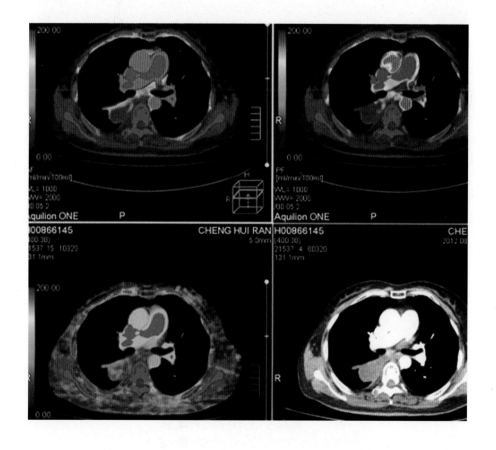

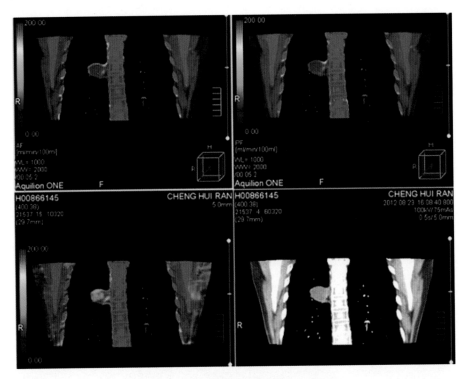

图 4 - 2 - 4　横断面及冠状面 CT 灌注图

病变为乏血供，肺循环、支气管循环血供均很弱，肺循环稍占优势

【病例3】

患者，女，22 岁。咳嗽、咳痰 1 年，加重 1 个月，发热（体温最高达 39.2℃）纳差 5d。临床诊断：空洞型肺结核。CT 显示见图 4 - 2 - 5，图 4 - 2 - 6。

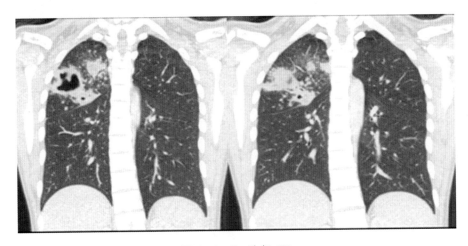

图 4 - 2 - 5　胸部 CT

右肺中上叶可见不规则空洞伴周围卫星灶

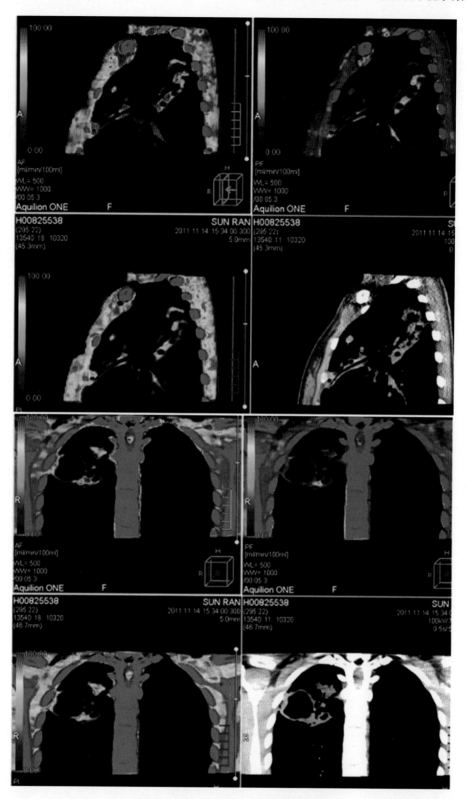

图 4-2-6　CT 灌注矢状面及冠状面图

右上肺病灶以肺动脉供血为主

【病例4】

男，74 岁。患者主诉咳嗽、咳痰、乏力、盗汗、消瘦半年余。CT 显示见图 4 - 2 - 7，图 4 - 2 - 8。

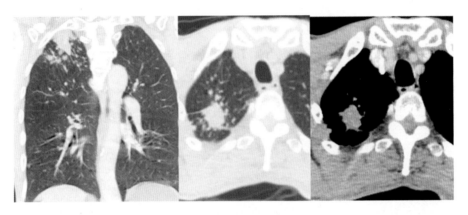

图 4 - 2 - 7　胸部 CT

右肺尖可见一结节状高密度影，边界可见毛刺，内见少许斑点样钙化，周围肺野可见卫星灶。增强扫描未见明显强化

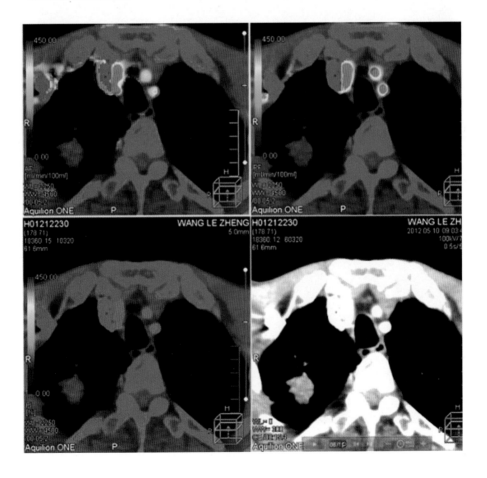

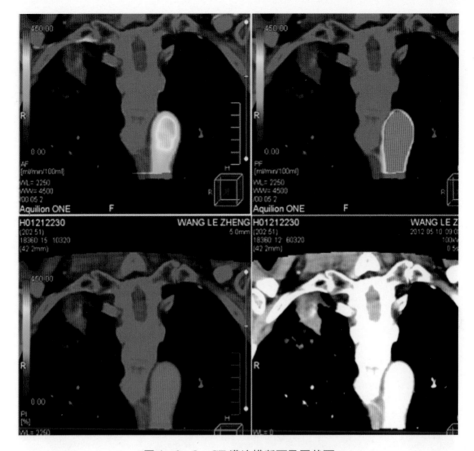

图 4 - 2 - 8　CT 灌注横断面及冠状面

右肺尖结节灶呈少许肺动脉供血，基本没有体循环供血

二、结核合并体动脉 - 肺动脉瘘

【病例 1】

男，42 岁。结核病史 3 年，咯血 2 周，右上肺结核伴空洞形成。CT 显示见图 4 - 2 - 9，图 4 - 2 - 10。

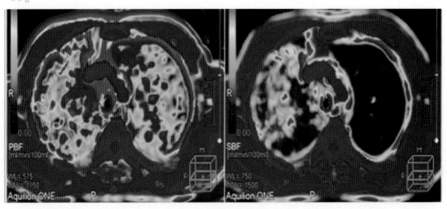

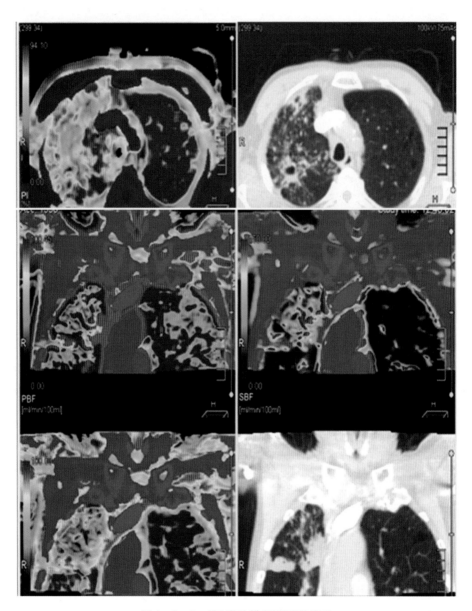

图 4 – 2 – 9 CT 灌注横断面及冠状面

右上肺病灶间肺实质呈明显体动脉血流灌注，灌注指数图（Perfusion index，PI）左肺呈较均匀红色，肺动脉血流灌注占绝对优势，为正常肺实质灌注表现，而右上肺肺实质灌注指数明显下降，提示支气管动脉（体动脉）—肺动脉瘘

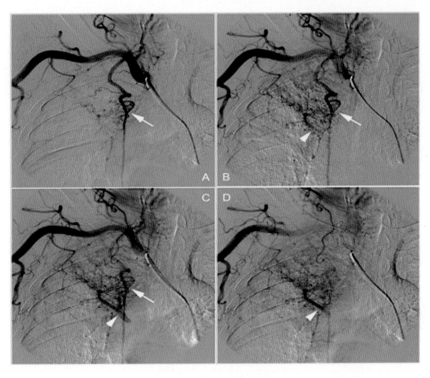

图 4 - 2 - 10　DSA 造影

右上肺灌注异常部位存在体动脉—肺动脉瘘：箭示胸廓内动脉分支，箭头示右上肺动脉，其间瘘形成至肺动脉及远端肺实质染色显影

【病例2】

男，37 岁。结核病史 4 年，咯血 1 周，右肺散在结核灶。CT 显示见图 4 - 2 - 11，图 4 - 2 - 12。

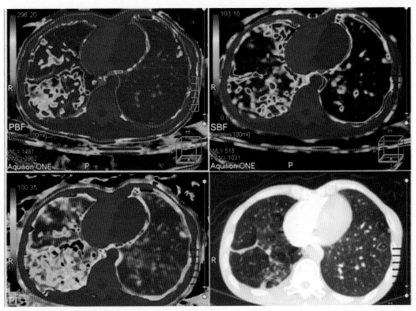

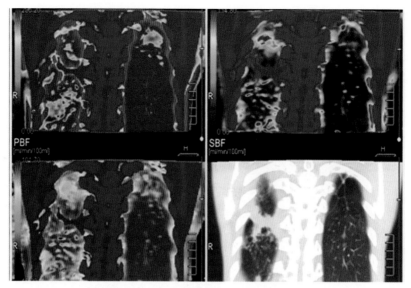

图 4 - 2 - 11　CT 灌注横断面及冠状面

右肺上叶及下叶病灶间肺实质体动脉血流灌注较正常（对侧）升高，灌注指数图（Perfusion index，PI）左肺呈较均匀红色，肺动脉血流灌注占绝对优势，为正常肺实质灌注表现，而右上肺及下肺实质灌注指数明显下降，提示支气管动脉（体动脉）—肺动脉瘘

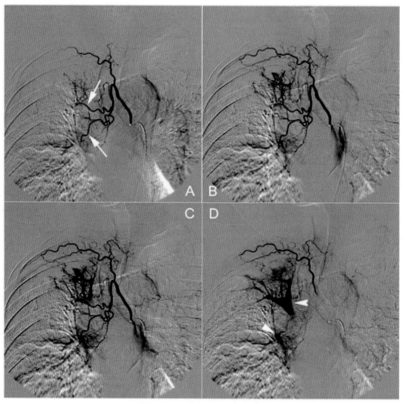

图 4 - 2 - 12　DSA 造影

右上肺及下肺灌注异常部位存在体动脉—肺动脉瘘：箭示支气管动脉分支，箭头示右上肺动脉及右下肺动脉，其间瘘形成至肺动脉及远端肺实质染色显影伴不规则迂曲血管显影

【病例 3】

女，47 岁。结核病史 5 年，咯血 3 周，左肺结核。CT 显示见图 4 - 2 - 13，图 4 - 2 - 14。

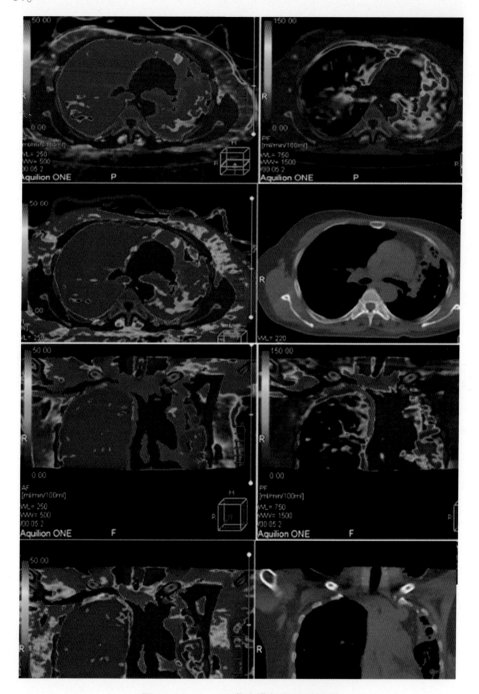

图 4 - 2 - 13　CT 灌注横断面及冠状面

左肺上叶病灶及病灶间肺实质体动脉血流灌注明显升高，灌注指数图（Perfusion index，PI）右肺呈较均匀红色，肺动脉血流灌注占绝对优势，为基本正常肺实质灌注表现，而右上肺肺实质灌注指数明显下降，提示支气管动脉（体动脉）—肺动脉瘘

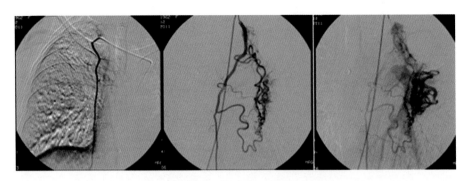

图 4 - 2 - 14 DSA 造影

证实左上肺灌注异常部位存在体动脉—肺动脉瘘：中间及右侧图片为左侧胸廓内动脉造影，证实分支通过迂曲血管团（瘘）与左肺动脉沟通，至左肺动脉及远端肺实质染色显影；左侧图片为右侧胸廓内动脉造影，未见明显异常

第三节 肺内其他病变的双重供血 CT 灌注

一、炎性假瘤

【病例 1】

男，53 岁。体检发现左上肺占位，临床诊断（结合病理表现）为炎性假瘤。CT 显示见图 4 - 3 - 1，图 4 - 3 - 2。

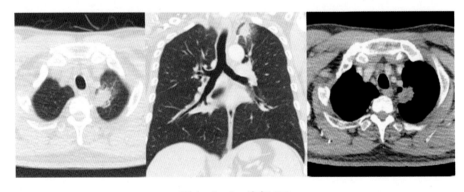

图 4 - 3 - 1 胸部 CT

左肺尖可见一结节状高密度影，边界毛糙，可见毛刺影，其内密度欠均

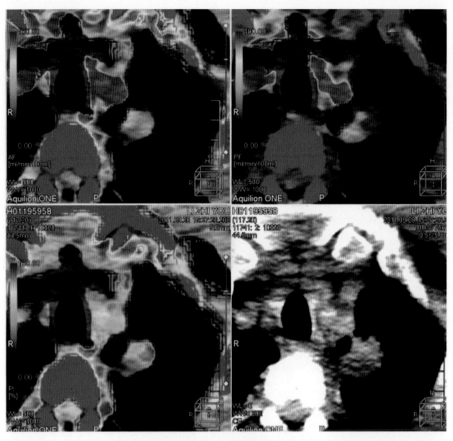

图 4 - 3 - 2　CT 灌注横断面
病变以肺动脉供血占优势

【病例 2】

女，51 岁。慢性咳嗽 1 年余，胸片发现左肺占位，临床诊断（结合病理表现）为炎性假瘤。CT 显示见图 4 - 3 - 3，图 4 - 3 - 4。

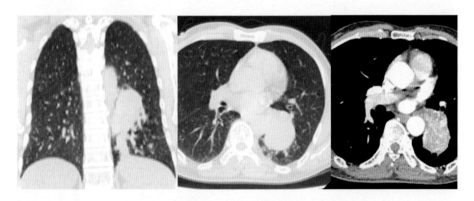

图 4 - 3 - 3　胸部 CT
左肺下叶可见一团块状高密度影，左肺下叶背段及基底段支气管均变窄，病变边缘较光整，病灶呈明显强化，强化不均匀，远端肺野可见少许阻塞性肺炎改变

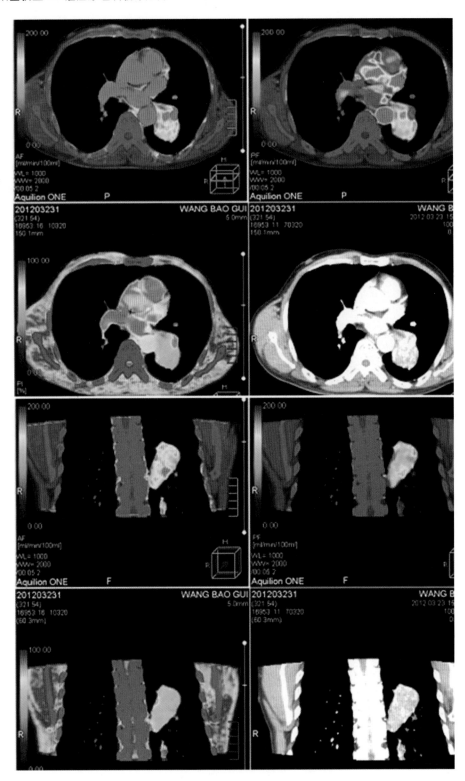

图 4 - 3 - 4　横断面及冠状面 CT 灌注

病变血供较丰富，为肺动脉、支气管动脉双重供血，肺循环血供略占优势

【病例3】

　　患者，女，28 岁。发热、咳嗽、胸闷，胸片发现右肺占位，临床诊断（结合病理表现）为炎性假瘤。CT 显示见图 4 - 3 - 5，图 4 - 3 - 6。

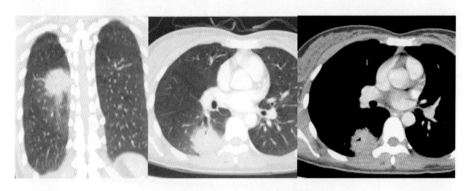

图 4 - 3 - 5　胸部 CT

右肺下叶背段可见一团片状高密度影，边界欠清晰，似伴细毛刺，邻近胸膜稍增厚。增强扫描明显强化

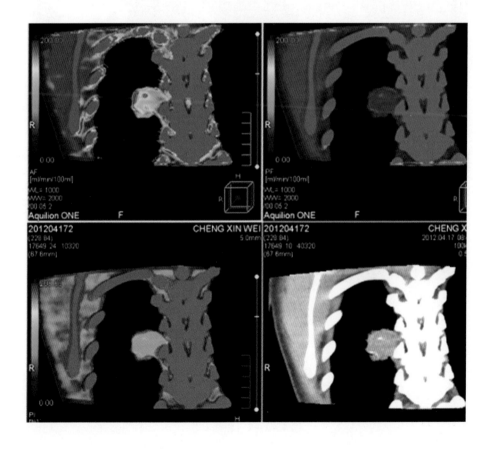

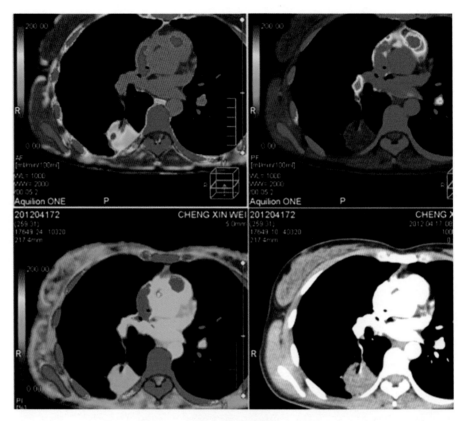

图 4 - 3 - 6　冠状面及横断面 CT 灌注

病变以肺循环供血占绝对优势，几乎没有体循环血供

【病例 4】

患者，男，63 岁。咳嗽、胸闷 3 个月。CT 显示见图 4 - 3 - 7，图 4 - 3 - 8。

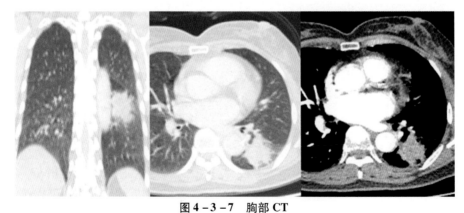

图 4 - 3 - 7　胸部 CT

左肺下叶背段分叶状肿块，增强扫描呈较明显强化

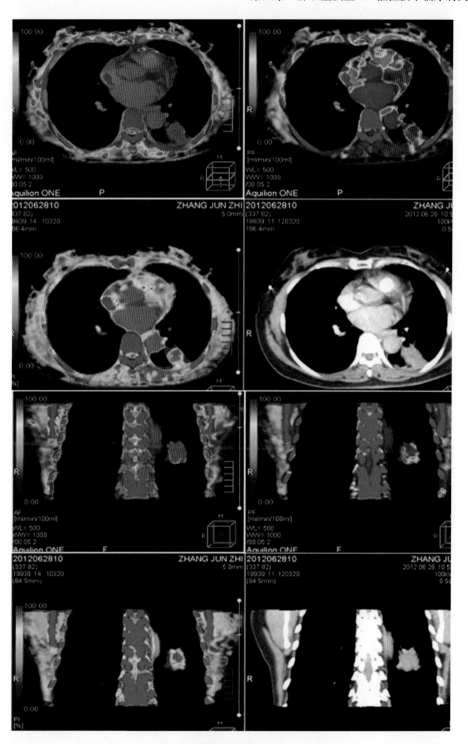

图 4 – 3 – 8　横断面及冠状面 CT 灌注

病变以肺循环供血占绝对优势，病灶中央几乎没有体循环血供，病灶外周见少许体循环供血

【病例5】

患者，男，70岁。因"感冒"症状持续1周到当地医院就诊，行胸片检查提示右上肺占位，进一步行胸部 CT 检查。CT 显示见图 4 - 3 - 9，图 4 - 3 - 10。

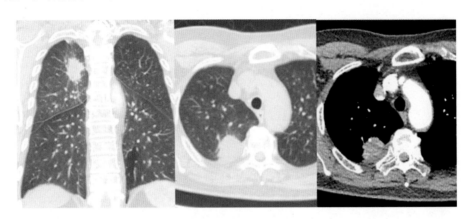

图 4 - 3 - 9　胸部 CT

右肺上叶后段可见一大小约 2.7 cm × 3.3 cm 软组织肿块影，浅分叶状，内密度较均匀，局部与胸膜有牵拉；增强扫描呈中等程度强化

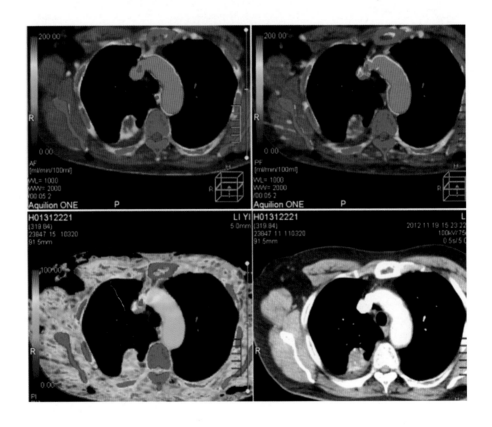

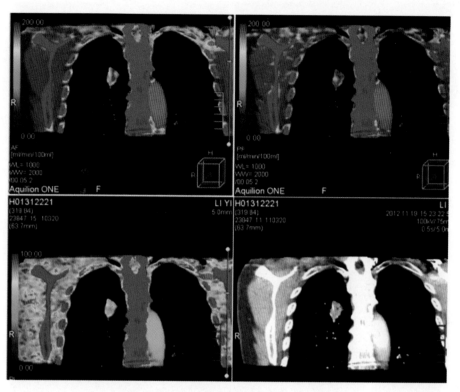

图4-3-10 横断面及冠状面CT灌注
病灶由肺循环和支气管循环双重供血，以肺循环血供略占优势

二、机化性肺炎

【病例1】

女性，56岁。慢性咳嗽半年余，胸片示右下肺病灶，病理诊断为肺组织慢性炎。CT显示见图4-3-11至图4-3-16。

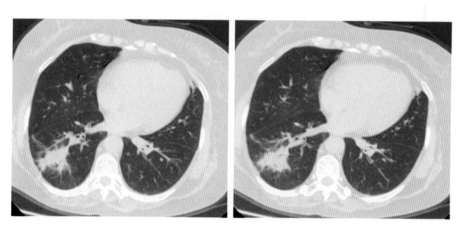

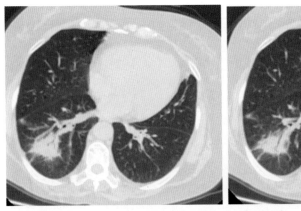
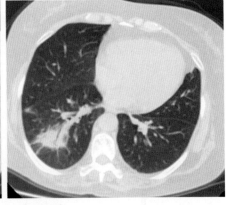

图 4 - 3 - 11　CT 横断面

右下肺团片状高密度灶，伴邻近胸膜牵拉

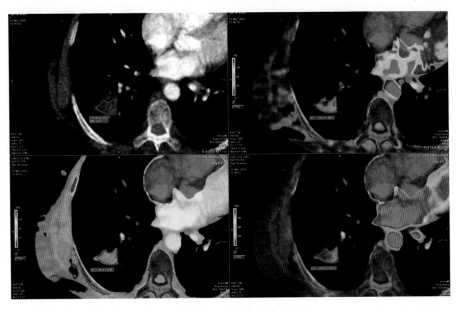

图 4 - 3 - 12　横断面灌注图

肺动脉血流量（pulmonary flow，PF）、支气管动脉血流量（bronchial flow，BF）、灌注指数（perfusion index，PI）分别为：168.6 ml/min/100 ml、69.9 ml/min/100 ml、71.2%

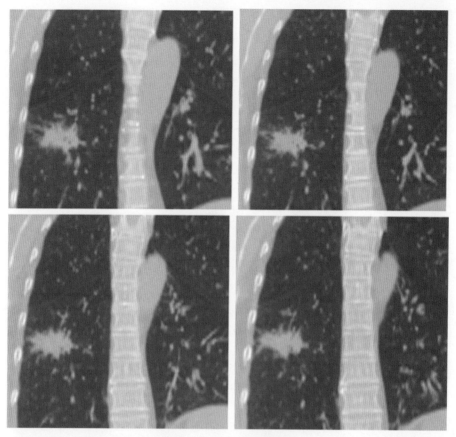

图 4 - 3 - 13　CT 冠状面

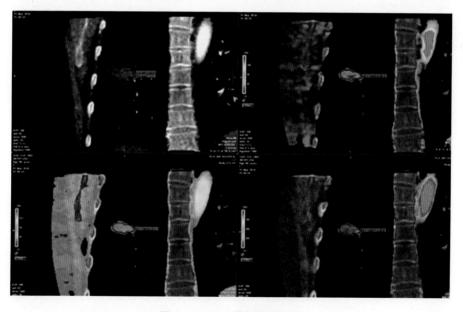

图 4 - 3 - 14　横断面灌注图

肺动脉血流量（pulmonary flow，PF）、支气管动脉血流量（bronchial flow，BF）、灌注指数（perfusion index，PI）分别为：151.8 ml/min/100 ml、68.8 ml/min/100 ml、70.2%

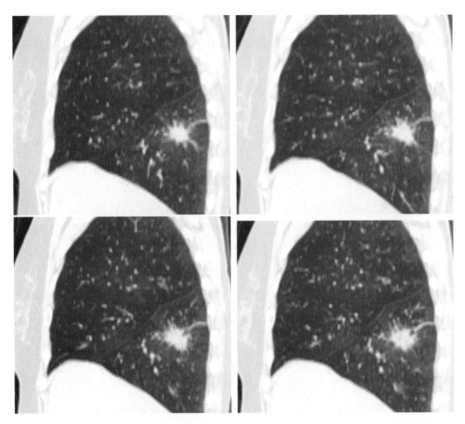

图 4 – 3 – 15   CT 矢状面

不规则形病灶位于右肺下叶背段

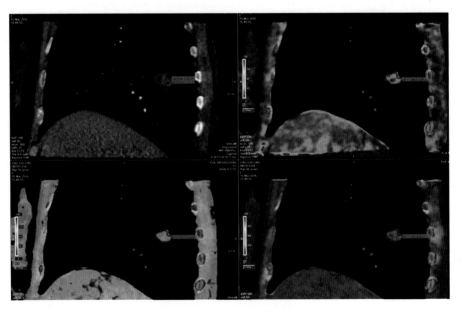

图 4 – 3 – 16   矢状面灌注图

肺动脉血流量（pulmonary flow，PF）、支气管动脉血流量（bronchial flow，BF）、灌注指数
（perfusion index，PI）分别为：150.7 ml/min/100 ml、64.5 ml/min/100 ml、70.3%

【病例2】

女，29岁。咳嗽1个月，胸片示左肺病灶，病理诊断左下肺慢性炎伴急性炎及多量坏死。CT显示见图4-3-17至图4-3-22。

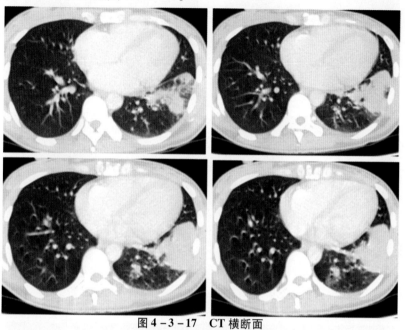

图4-3-17　CT横断面

左下肺团片状病灶

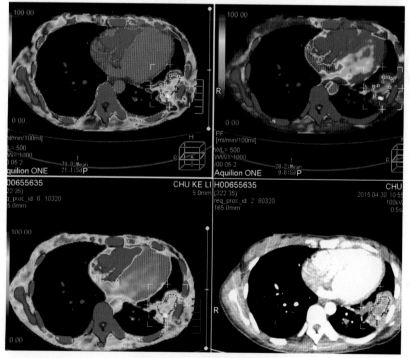

图4-3-18　横断面灌注图

肺动脉血流量（pulmonary flow，PF）、支气管动脉血流量（bronchial flow，BF）、灌注指数（perfusion index，PI）分别为：59.2 ml/min/100 ml、37.2 ml/min/100 ml、60.7%

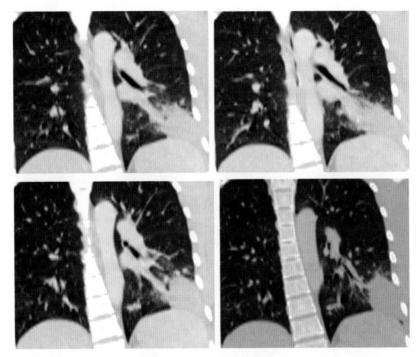

图 4 - 3 - 19 CT 冠状面

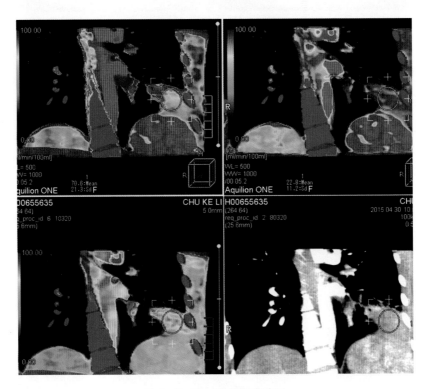

图 4 - 3 - 20 冠状面灌注图

肺动脉血流量（pulmonary flow，PF）、支气管动脉血流量（bronchial flow，BF）、灌注指数（perfusion index，PI）分别为：59.4 ml/min/100 ml、44.9 ml/min/100 ml、55.9%

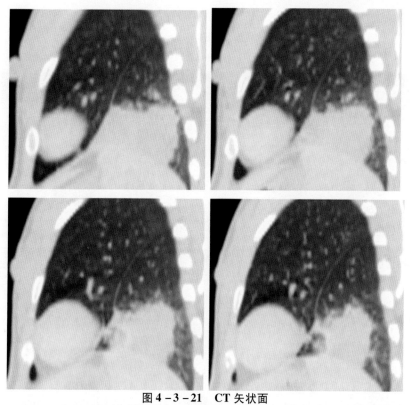

图 4 - 3 - 21　CT 矢状面

病灶位于左膈面上方，呈团片状，邻近斜裂胸膜有牵拉

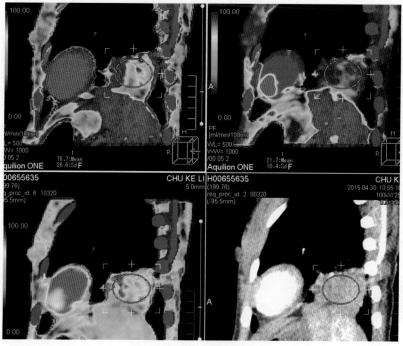

图 4 - 3 - 22　冠状面灌注图

肺动脉血流量（pulmonary flow，PF）、支气管动脉血流量（bronchial flow，BF）、灌注指数（perfusion index，PI）分别为：58.7 ml/min/100 ml、48.7 ml/min/100 ml、54.0%

【病例3】

男，67岁。胸闷1个月余，胸片示左上肺病灶，病理诊断为左上少许支气管黏膜及肺组织慢性炎。CT显示见图4-3-23至图4-3-27。

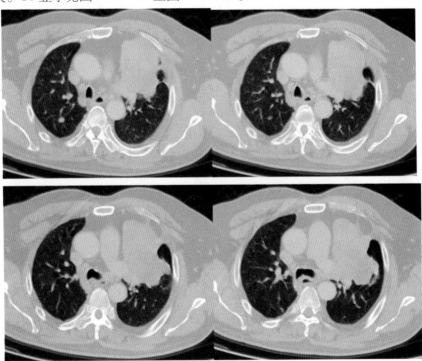

图4-3-23　CT横断面

左上肺团片状病灶

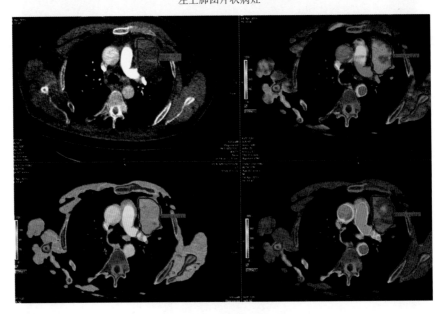

图4-3-24　横断面灌注图

肺动脉血流量（pulmonary flow，PF）、支气管动脉血流量（bronchial flow，BF）、灌注指数（perfusion index，PI）分别为：71.5 ml/min/100 ml、63.6 ml/min/100 ml、55.8%

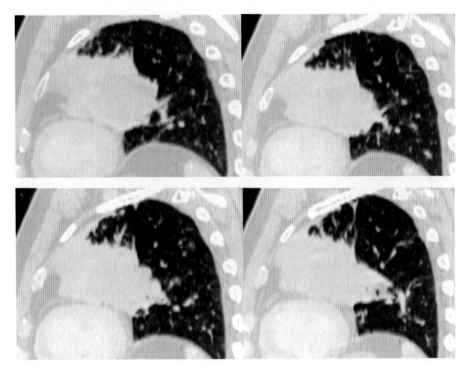

图 4 – 3 – 25　CT 矢状面

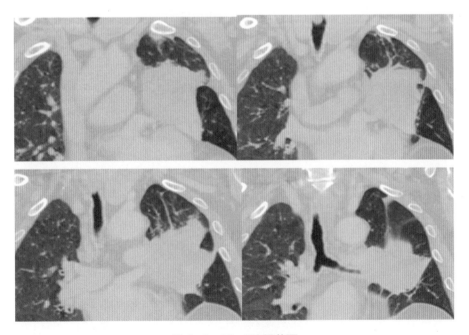

图 4 – 3 – 26　CT 冠状面

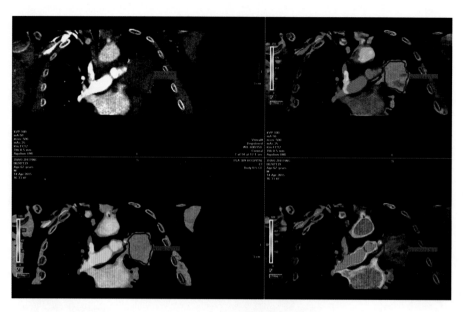

图 4 - 3 - 27　冠状面灌注图

肺动脉血流量（pulmonary flow，PF）、支气管动脉血流量（bronchial flow，BF）、灌注指数（perfusion index，PI）分别为：81.0 ml/min/100 ml、79.5 ml/min/100 ml、50.7%

附　录

CT 灌注相关研究论著

Eur Radiol (2012) 22:1665–1671
DOI 10.1007/s00330-012-2414-5

CHEST

Lung cancer perfusion: can we measure pulmonary and bronchial circulation simultaneously?

Xiaodong Yuan · Jing Zhang · Guokun Ao ·
Changbin Quan · Yuan Tian · Hong Li

Received: 16 October 2011 / Revised: 26 December 2011 / Accepted: 4 January 2012 / Published online: 14 March 2012
© European Society of Radiology 2012

Abstract

Objective To describe a new CT perfusion technique for assessing the dual blood supply in lung cancer and present the initial results.

Methods This study was approved by the institutional review board. A CT protocol was developed, and a dual-input CT perfusion (DI-CTP) analysis model was applied and evaluated regarding the blood flow fractions in lung tumours. The pulmonary trunk and the descending aorta were selected as the input arteries for the pulmonary circulation and the bronchial circulation respectively. Pulmonary flow (PF), bronchial flow (BF), and a perfusion index (PI, = PF/ (PF + BF)) were calculated using the maximum slope method. After written informed consent was obtained, 13 consecutive subjects with primary lung cancer underwent DI-CTP.

Results Perfusion results are as follows: PF, 13.45± 10.97 ml/min/100 ml; BF, 48.67±28.87 ml/min/100 ml; PI, 21 %±11 %. BF is significantly larger than PF, $P < 0.001$. There is a negative correlation between the tumour volume and perfusion index ($r=0.671$, $P=0.012$).

Conclusion The dual-input CT perfusion analysis method can be applied successfully to lung tumours. Initial results demonstrate a dual blood supply in primary lung cancer, in which the systemic circulation is dominant, and that the proportion of the two circulation systems is moderately dependent on tumour size.

Key Points

- *A new CT perfusion technique can assess lung cancer's dual blood supply.*
- *A dual blood supply was confirmed with dominant bronchial circulation in lung cancer.*
- *The proportion of the two circulations is moderately dependent on tumour size.*
- *This new technique may benefit the management of lung cancer.*

Keywords Lung cancer · Dual blood supply · Perfusion CT · Area detector · Computed tomography

Abbreviations

DI-CTP	Dual-input CT perfusion
PA	Pulmonary artery
BA	Bronchial artery
TDCs	Time density curves
PF	Pulmonary flow
BF	Bronchial flow
PI = PF/(PF + BF)	Perfusion index

X. Yuan · G. Ao (✉) · C. Quan · Y. Tian · H. Li
Department of Radiology,
The 309th Hospital of Chinese People's Liberation Army,
17 Heishanhu Road, Haidian District,
Beijing 100091, People's Republic of China
e-mail: aoguokun309@163.com

J. Zhang
Department of Radiology, Tongji Hospital of Tongji University,
389 Xincun Road,
Shanghai 200065, People's Republic of China

Introduction

Recently perfusion CT has become a major imaging technique for assessing tumour angiogenesis and the therapeutic effect of anti-angiogenic drugs because of the accessibility of the technology and its ability to provide quantification of

Eur Radiol (2012) 22:1665–1671

the haemodynamics of lesions with mass effect [1, 2]. Previously lung cancer CT perfusion analysis was performed using the single input perfusion model with the input artery as either the PA or the aorta (as a substitute for BA). There is some debate as to the origin and/or the proportion of blood supply in lung cancer [3–7]. If one considers the BA as the only or dominant blood supply in lung cancer, the aorta will be chosen as the input artery and vice versa.

In the early 1970s it was discovered through necropsy that lung tumours have a dual vascular supply [8]; however in vivo quantification of the dual blood supply in lung cancer with CT perfusion has not been possible due in large part to the limitations of the technology. The respective proportion of the dual blood supply in lung tumours has not been previously described with CT perfusion, to our knowledge. The quantification of the dual blood supply to lung tumours and the relative proportions of each can potentially aid in the management of lung cancer.

We developed a new CT perfusion technique for measuring the dual blood supply in lung tumours and performed this technique prospectively in 13 consecutive subjects with bronchogenic carcinoma.

Materials and methods

Dual-input CT perfusion imaging technique

Before the examination, all patients underwent breath training to ensure that they could hold their breath for the entire perfusion process (approximately 30 s). Shallow abdominal breathing was permitted at the end stage of acquisition in cases where the patient was unable to hold their breath for the entire period of CT data acquisition. Two 20-gauge intravenous catheters were placed, one in each antecubital vein.

Before the perfusion CT acquisition, an unenhanced helical CT of the entire thorax was performed to determine the location of the lesion with mass effect. Dynamic CT perfusion was performed using a 320-detector row CT (Aquilion ONE, Toshiba Medical Systems, Otawara, Japan) with a z-axis coverage of 16 cm. With a dual-head power injector, 60 ml of non-ionic contrast medium with an iodine concentration of 370 mgI/ml (Iopromide, Bayer Schering, Berlin, Germany) was injected at a flow rate of 8 ml/s (4 ml/s on each side). Two seconds after the bolus injection, 15 intermittent low-dose volume acquisitions were made with 2-s intervals and without table movement (Fig. 1).

The dynamic CT protocol was performed with the following parameters: 80-kV tube voltage, 80-mA tube current, 0.5-s gantry rotation speed and 0.5-mm slice thickness. The 16-cm coverage included both the lung hilum and the lesion with mass effect.

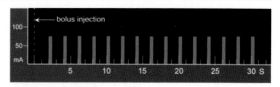

Fig. 1 The time sequence display of the perfusion CT with the Aquilion ONE system. Two seconds after the start of the bolus injection, 15 volume images were acquired with a 2-s interval. The breath-hold duration was approximately 30 s

The first two volumes were acquired before contrast medium arrived in the heart and served as a baseline. The duration of the breath hold was approximately 30 s. Image data sets were reconstructed with 0.5-mm slice thickness and 0.5-mm spacing, resulting in 320 images per volume and a total of 4,800 images for the entire perfusion data set.

Data Post-processing and analysis

Post-processing was performed using perfusion software available on the CT equipment (Body Perfusion, Toshiba Medical Systems, Otawara, Japan). The first step is volume registration. The registration is performed to correct for motion between the dynamic volumes and creates a registered volume series. The registered volumes were then loaded into the body perfusion analysis software.

Rectangular ROIs (mean area 1.0 cm^2) were manually placed in the pulmonary artery trunk and the aorta at the level of the hilum to generate the TDCs representing the PA input function and the BA input function respectively. An elliptical ROI was placed in the left atrium, and the peak time of the left atrium TDC was used to differentiate pulmonary circulation (before the peak time point) and bronchial circulation (after the peak time point; Fig. 2). A freehand ROI was drawn to encompass the lesion with mass effect to generate the TDC of the contrast medium's first-pass attenuation in the tissue of the tumour. The perfusion analysis range was set from 0 HU to 150 HU to restrict the perfusion analysis to soft tissue regions only and to ignore lung parenchyma and bone. Finally, 512×512 matrix colour-coded maps of PF, BF, and PI (PI = PF/ (PF + BF)) were produced automatically. For each lesion, measurements were repeated on all relevant 5.0-mm axial slices and then averaged to calculate the final value. Tumour volume (size) was measured on commercial software (organ selection, Vitrea version 6.0, Vital Images, Minnetonka, MN, USA).

Study population

Thirteen consecutive patients were included in the study (9 men and 4 women; mean age, 52 years; range, 41–65 years),

⁂ Springer

Eur Radiol (2012) 22:1665–1671

Fig. 2 Time-density curves (TDCs) of pulmonary artery (PA), bronchial artery (BA), left atrium and lung tumour. The vertical dashed line indicates the peak enhancement time point of the left atrium, which is located between the two peaks of the PA and the BA; therefore, it is used to distinguish between pulmonary and bronchial circulation. The TDC of the lung tumour had two ascending slopes representing pulmonary and bronchial circulation respectively. The latter was much steeper than the former, which suggests that bronchial circulation was dominant in this case

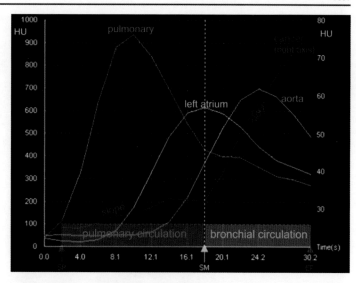

all with a solitary pulmonary nodule/mass pathologically confirmed as bronchogenic carcinoma (6 squamous cell carcinoma, 2 adeno-squamous carcinoma, 3 adenocarcinoma, 2 small cell lung carcinoma) through CT-guided puncture biopsy or bronchoscopy biopsy or surgical resection within the 2 weeks before/after the perfusion CT. They were all untreated before the perfusion CT and enrolled prospectively into the study. The study had institutional review board approval, and written informed consent was obtained from all patients, which included information about the radiation exposure of the CT examinations. Exclusion criteria were pregnancy, previous reactions to iodinated contrast media and dyspnoea.

The radiation dose of both the dynamic and helical CT was calculated from the dose–length product (DLP) listed in the exposure summary sheet generated by the CT equipment and multiplied by a factor of 0.014 [9].

Statistical analysis

Statistical analysis was performed using commercially available software (SPSS, V13.0). Paired Student's t-test was used to compare PF with BF. Tumour size correlated with the perfusion index. A *P* value lower than 0.05 was considered to indicate a significant difference.

Results

Five patients adopted shallow abdominal breathing because of hypoxia at the end stage of the perfusion CT. All patients showed good compliance with the CT perfusion procedure despite the relatively high injection rate of contrast agent

and the slightly long breath-hold duration of 30 s. No severe adverse events occurred.

Perfusion parameters were visualised by colour maps and fused onto the original axial CT images. Representative perfusion colour maps are shown in Figs. 3 and 4. Quantitative perfusion parameters of the 13 primary lung cancers derived from DI-CTP are listed in Table 1. Mean tumour volume was 32.98 cm³, ranging from 5.64 to 69.91 cm³. The dynamic perfusion protocol was identical for all 13 cases with the CT dose DLP=324.8 mGy. cm or 4.55 mSv (k=0.014).

Discussion

The lungs have a dual vascular blood supply, the pulmonary circulation and the bronchial circulation. The pulmonary circulation is dominant in the total blood supply volume. Although the bronchial circulation only accounts for a small amount of the total blood volume supply in normal lung tissue, it is crucial for maintaining airway and lung function [10]. The bronchial circulation is more transitional under pathological conditions and plays an important role in many lung diseases, especially in lung cancer where there is some debate regarding its role and importance in terms of the tumour blood supply and therefore tumour growth and biology. Measurement of the two circulations is meaningful both physiologically and pathologically.

The new perfusion technique described here is potentially valuable for both differential diagnosis and treatment planning:

1. PI as a new parameter derived from DI-CTP has the potential to differentiate lung cancer from some benign

1668   Eur Radiol (2012) 22:1665–1671

Fig. 3 Example 1: Coloured parametric maps in a 45-year-old male patient with a right inferior lung nodule pathologically confirmed as adenocarcinoma (arrow). Adjacent atelectasis was revealed by abundant pulmonary flow (PF) and a relatively high perfusion index (PI; arrow head). The tumour is undersized in our cohort and demonstrates near equilibrium between pulmonary and bronchial circulation at this level

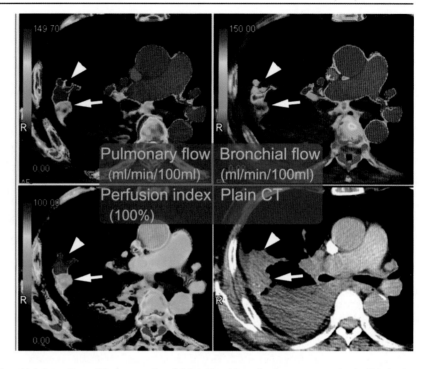

lesions such as atelectasis, which has a larger PI physiologically (Fig. 3);

2. Of the 13 subjects in the current study the BA is the dominant blood supply with more or less from the PA

Fig. 4 Example 2: Coloured parametric maps in the coronal plane in a 53-year-old male patient with squamous cell carcinoma located in the left inferior lung. The perfusion is heterogeneous throughout the tumour. Bronchial circulation is globally dominant even though the peripheral region of the tumour is mainly fed by the PA (arrowhead)

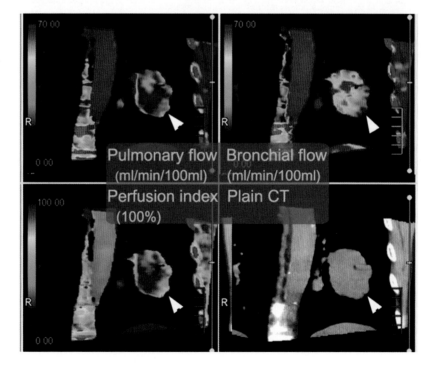

Eur Radiol (2012) 22:1665–1671

Table 1 Perfusion results

Perfusion parameters	n	Mean	SD	95% CI		Paired t-test
				Lower	Upper	
PF (ml/min/100 mL)	13	13.45	10.97	6.83	20.08	$t=4.997$
BF (ml/min/100 ml)	13	48.67	28.87	31.22	66.11	$P<0.001$
PI (100%)	13	0.21	0.11	0.14	0.27	

Footnote: pulmonary flow (PF), bronchial flow (BF), perfusion index (PI)

(Table 1, Fig. 5), which implies that if interventional therapy is to be performed on these patients, then trans-pulmonary artery treatment could be considered as well as trans-bronchial artery treatment, especially for those with abundant PF (Fig. 3). Therefore this technique may benefit the treatment planning of lung cancer. Although the systemic circulation is dominant (accounting for more than half of the total tumour blood supply volume) in every subject in our cohort, PI, which indicates the proportion of the two circulations, varies from subject to subject. This is partially dependent on tumour volume (Fig. 6); for a few tumours that are of small volume, the PI is close to 50%, suggesting near equilibrium between pulmonary and systemic circulation. Tumours that are larger in size demonstrate a larger proportion of systemic circulation. From a different perspective, the correlation between PI and tumour volume may be hinting that as bronchogenic carcinoma develops, the systemic circulation increases and eventually becomes the dominant

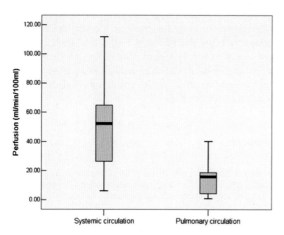

Fig. 5 Box plot of systemic and pulmonary circulation. Systemic circulation is more dominant than the pulmonary circulation in bronchogenic carcinoma. Systemic circulation also varies within a wider range than pulmonary circulation

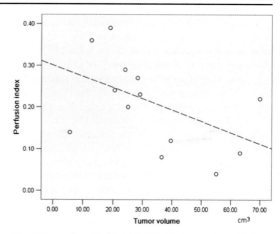

Fig. 6 Scatter plot of perfusion index and tumour volume. Negative correlation between tumour size and perfusion index is revealed: Pearson's correlation coefficient is 0.671 (moderate correlation), which is significant at the 0.05 level ($P=0.012$)

blood supply to the tumour. This gives DI-CTP the potential to determine disease progression.

In addition to the BA, systemic circulation in the lung can also originate from intercostal arteries, subclavian arteries, the internal thoracic artery, inferior phrenic artery, etc. As they all arise from the aorta, the TDC of the aorta is used as the input function for systemic circulation when performing DI-CTP analysis in lung tumours. The feeding artery of the systemic circulation is described as the bronchial artery in this analysis and its measurements were recorded as BF regardless of the actual origin of the systemic blood supply.

The concept of using two feeding vessels as input functions for the maximum slope analysis method to calculate the dual blood supply in one organ was originally described by Miles et al. to calculate hepatic perfusion [11]. The abdominal aorta and the portal vein are selected as the dual-input vessels; the peak time point of the spleen enhancement is used to differentiate hepatic artery circulation and portal vein circulation. Based on the maximum slope method, blood flow by the two vessels can be calculated as the maximum slopes of the tissue enhancement divided by the peak values of the two input vessels' enhancement [12]. Similarly in our study, PA and BA were selected as the two input vessels, the peak enhancement time point of the left atrium was used to separate the PA and BA circulation. Figure 2 demonstrates this time point located between the two peaks of the PA and BA TDCs, so it is an appropriate boundary for differentiating between these two circulations. When the left atrium is not included in the 16-cm coverage, the boundary can be set manually between the two peaks, theoretically with the same results.

🖄 Springer

Eur Radiol (2012) 22:1665–1671

Considering the left atrium lies functionally between the pulmonary circulation and the bronchial circulation, its peak enhancement time was chosen to divide the tissue TDC into a 'pulmonary part' and a 'bronchial part'. This was used in all 13 cases. The software then determined the maximum slope of the 'pulmonary part' and the 'bronchial part' separately and then calculated the respective blood flow. This is the key point. In regard to Fig. 2, the tissue TDC showed a clear turning point coinciding with the left atrium peak time thus supporting our choice to use the left atrium peak time. Some cases in our study cohort demonstrated a plateau between slope 2 and slope 1, so there was no obvious turning point between them. In these cases the peak of the enhancement of the left atrium occurred within the plateau, making it a good point for dividing the two circulations.

When a single input CT perfusion technique was employed in lung cancer perfusion analysis, according to the theory of the maximum slope method, the dominant circulation will be calculated and the secondary circulation is ignored. When considering Fig. 2, for example, slope 2 will be considered as the circulation of the tumour, while slope 1 will be ignored. That is to say results concerning lung cancer perfusion to date have effectively only measured that from the bronchial circulation. In this sense other studies may have systematically underestimated lung cancer perfusion owing to ignoring the dual blood supply.

The DI-CTP adopted in the present study is based on the maximum slope method, which only takes into account the initial upslope of the tissue TDC, and the input vessel's peak enhancement value. Therefore the duration of the acquisition can be shorter than when the deconvolution method is used for analysis, which utilises both the ascending and the descending portions of the TDC. A shorter acquisition time will result in a lower radiation dose. However, the maximum slope analysis method has the following limitations:

1. The blood volume (BV) and the mean transit time (MTT) cannot be generated directly by the maximum slope method;
2. Contrast agent was injected through bilateral antecubital veins to achieve a high flow rate, which is required by the perfusion model hypothesis. Injection rates of between 5 mLl/s and 10 ml/s are required by the maximum slope method owing to its theoretical assumption that the tissue maximum slope enhancement is reached before venous drainage begins. For a fixed total contrast agent volume, a higher injection rate means shorter injection duration, resulting in sharper shapes of the TDCs of the two input arteries, therefore leading to less overlap in the phase domain between these two circulations (Fig.2) [13]. A large overlap could somewhat undermine the reliability of measurements in DI-CTP, especially for the assessment of systemic circulation due to residual perfusion from the pulmonary circulation. Besides, a high flow rate may also be of benefit by maximising tissue enhancement and so improving the signal-to-noise ratio [14].

Until now, the pulmonary and bronchial circulation in lung cancer tumours has not been assessed simultaneously, which is mainly due to the limited coverage along the z-axis of CT systems with less than 320 detector rows. With the Aquilion ONE's 16-cm volume imaging, coverage along the z-axis easily covers more than half of an adult's lung. The hilum and lesion can usually be included in a single volume. Therefore the PA, the aorta, the left atrium and the lesion studied are included in one temporally uniform acquisition, which makes the DI-CTP analysis method possible in lung tumours.

An intrinsic limitation of perfusion CT is the radiation exposure, which increases with tube voltage, tube current and the number of CT volume exposures. In order to keep the overall radiation dose within the range of clinical utility, we reduced the kV and mA in the perfusion CT so that the overall dose (including the localisation imaging) equals approximately the same dose as a triphasic abdominal imaging procedure [15, 16]. Additionally, because of its shorter acquisition time we utilised the maximum slope method rather than the deconvolution method to calculate the perfusion, therefore keeping to the target dose of our perfusion protocol. Post-processing of volumetric DI-CTP takes about 5–10 min with volume registration. At present it may not be suitable for emergency use. In addition, the relatively small sample size and potential heterogeneity of lesions in our study may reduce the clinical significance of our primary findings. Population-based research is warranted to further determine the clinical utility of this method.

In conclusion, a dual-input perfusion analysis technique and imaging protocol for lung tumours has been described. It demonstrates two main features: firstly, that there is a dual blood supply pattern in primary lung cancer, of which the systemic bronchial circulation is usually dominant; secondly, that the proportion of the two circulations is moderately dependent on tumour size.

References

1. Goh V, Halligan S, Daley F et al (2008) Colorectal tumor vascularity: quantitative assessment with multidetector CT—do tumor perfusion measurements reflect angiogenesis? Radiology 249:510–517
2. Fournier LS, Oudard S, Thiam R et al (2010) Metastatic renal carcinoma: evaluation of antiangiogenic therapy with dynamic contrast-enhanced CT. Radiology 256:511–518
3. Tacelli N, Remy-Jardin M, Copin MC et al (2010) Assessment of non-small cell lung cancer perfusion: pathologic-CT correlation in 15 patients. Radiology 257:863–871

Springer

Eur Radiol (2012) 22:1665–1671

4. Milne EN, Zerhouni AE (1987) Blood supply of pulmonary metastases. J Thoracic Imaging 2:15–23

5. Kiessling F, Boese J, Corvinus C et al (2004) Perfusion CT in patients with advanced bronchial carcinomas: a novel chance for characterization and treatment monitoring? Eur Radiol 14:1226–1233

6. Viamonte M Jr (1965) Angiographic evaluation of lung neoplasms. Radiol Clin North Am 3:529–542

7. Hellekant C (1979) Bronchial angiography and intraarterial chemotherapy with mitomycin-C in bronchogenic carcinoma: anatomy, technique, complications. Acta Radiol Diagn (Stockh) 20:478–496

8. Milne EN (1967) Circulation of primary and metastatic pulmonary neoplasms: a postmortem microarteriographic study. Am J Roentgenol Radium Ther Nucl Med 100:603–619

9. Valentin J (2007) Managing patient dose in multi-detector computed tomography (MDCT). Ann ICRP 37:1–79

10. McCullagh A, Rosenthal M, Wanner A et al (2010) The bronchial circulation – worth a closer look: a review of the relationship between the bronchial vasculature and airway inflammation. Pediatr Pulmonol 45:1–13

11. Miles KA, Hayball MP, Dixon AK (1993) Functional images of hepatic perfusion obtained with dynamic CT. Radiology 188:405–411

12. Miles KA, Griffiths MR (2003) Perfusion CT: a worthwhile enhancement? Br J Radiol 76:220–231

13. Bae KT (2003) Peak contrast enhancement in CT and MR angiography: when does it occur and why? Pharmacokinetic study in a porcine model. Radiology 227:809–816

14. Miles KA (2003) Perfusion CT for the assessment of tumour vascularity: which protocol? Br J Radiol 76:S36–S42

15. Galanski M, Nagel HD, Stamm G (2007) Results of a federation inquiry 2005/2006: pediatric CT X-ray practice in Germany. Rofo 179:1110–1111

16. Tsai HY, Tung CJ, Yu CC, Tyan YS (2007) Survey of computed tomography scanners in Taiwan: dose descriptors, dose guidance levels, and effective doses. Med Phys 34:1234–1243

Springer

Eur Radiol (2013) 23:2469–2474
DOI 10.1007/s00330-013-2842-x

CHEST

Differentiation of malignant and benign pulmonary nodules with first-pass dual-input perfusion CT

Xiaodong Yuan · Jing Zhang · Changbin Quan · Jianxia Cao · Guokun Ao · Yuan Tian · Hong Li

Received: 17 November 2012 / Revised: 16 February 2013 / Accepted: 21 February 2013 / Published online: 22 June 2013
© European Society of Radiology 2013

Abstract

Objective To assess diagnostic performance of dual-input CT perfusion for distinguishing malignant from benign solitary pulmonary nodules (SPNs).

Methods Fifty-six consecutive subjects with SPNs underwent contrast-enhanced 320-row multidetector dynamic volume CT. The dual-input maximum slope CT perfusion analysis was employed to calculate the pulmonary flow (PF), bronchial flow (BF), and perfusion index (PI, = PF/(PF + BF)). Differences in perfusion parameters between malignant and benign tumours were assessed with histopathological diagnosis as the gold standard. Diagnostic value of the perfusion parameters was calculated using the receiver-operating characteristic (ROC) curve analysis.

Results Amongst 56 SPNs, statistically significant differences in all three perfusion parameters were revealed between malignant and benign tumours. The PI demonstrated the biggest difference between malignancy and benignancy: 0.30 ± 0.07 vs. 0.51 ± 0.13, $P<0.001$. The area under the PI ROC curve was 0.92, the largest of the three perfusion parameters, producing a sensitivity of 0.95, specificity of 0.83, positive likelihood ratio (+LR) of 5.59, and negative likelihood ratio (−LR) of 0.06 in identifying malignancy.

Conclusions The PI derived from the dual-input maximum slope CT perfusion analysis is a valuable biomarker for identifying malignancy in SPNs. PI may be potentially useful for lung cancer treatment planning and forecasting the therapeutic effect of radiotherapy treatment.

X. Yuan · C. Quan (✉) · J. Cao · G. Ao · Y. Tian · H. Li
Department of Radiology, the 309th Hospital of Chinese People's Liberation Army, 17 Heishanhu Road, Haidian District, Beijing 100091, People's Republic of China
e-mail: quanchangbin309@163.com

J. Zhang
Department of Radiology, Tongji Hospital of Tongji University, 389 Xincun Road, Shanghai 200065, People's Republic of China

Key Points
• *Modern CT equipment offers assessment of vascular parameters of solitary pulmonary nodules (SPNs)*
• *Dual vascular supply was investigated to differentiate malignant from benign SPNs.*
• *Different dual vascular supply patterns were found in malignant and benign SPNs.*
• *The perfusion index is a useful biomarker for differentiate malignancy from benignancy.*

Keywords Lung cancer · Solitary pulmonary nodule · 320-detector row CT · Dual-input maximum slope CT perfusion · ROC curve analysis

Abbreviations

DI-CTP	Dual-input maximum slope CT perfusion
SPN	Solitary pulmonary nodule
PA	Pulmonary artery
BA	Bronchial artery
TDCs	Time density curves
PF	Pulmonary flow
BF	Bronchial flow
(PI, = PF/(PF + BF))	Perfusion index
ROI	Region of interest
ROC curve	Receiver-operating characteristic curve
+LR	Positive likelihood ratio
−LR	Negative likelihood ratio

Introduction

In the early 1970s it was discovered through post-mortem microarteriography study that lung tumours have a dual vascular supply, i.e. the pulmonary circulation and the systemic circulation [1]. In vivo quantification of the dual blood

2470

Eur Radiol (2013) 23:2469–2474

supply in lung cancer by CT perfusion is now possible owing to the greater coverage along the z axis provided by the 320-row CT system [2]. Before this, perfusion or blood flow could only be measured within a coverage range limited by the detector width. Thus, the pulmonary artery usually could not be included in the perfusion imaging territory, and in most cases the aorta was selected as the input artery. The single-input maximum slope perfusion model was used to assess the lung tumour haemodynamics. The recent dynamic volume CT mode utilising the 320-row system (with 16-cm coverage in the z axis) makes it possible to include the pulmonary artery, the aorta, and the tumour studied in one gantry rotation without table movement. Then contrast-enhanced dynamic-volume acquisitions will simultaneously capture the pulmonary and systemic circulation input functions as well as the tumour's first-pass response function. It is then possible to assess the dual blood supply in lung tumours with the dual-input maximum slope analysis model.

Good management of the pulmonary nodules was supposed to reduce lung cancer mortality [3]. Differentiating malignant from benign SPNs when only conventional CT data are available is always a challenge for the radiologist because of the huge overlap in morphological findings between malignancy and benignity. With the development of multi-detector CT systems and the CT perfusion technique, tumour haemodynamics derived from perfusion measurements were used to help identify lung cancer [4, 5]. The single-input maximum slope analysis model was used for this purpose and proved helpful in the differential diagnosis between malignant and benign [6, 7]. Theoretically DI-CTP is more suitable for analysing lung tumour perfusion as it can estimate the pulmonary circulation and the bronchial or systemic circulation as separate perfusion parameters. To our knowledge, the pulmonary and the bronchial circulation (systemic circulation) has never been measured for discrimination between malignant and benign lung tumours. We hypothesise that quantification of the two circulations in SPNs might help to identify lung cancer. This prospective study was designed to determine the diagnostic value of DI-CTP in solitary pulmonary nodules for identifying lung cancer.

Materials and methods

Study population

The prospective study was approved by the institution's ethics committee. Written informed consent was obtained from all patients, and complete explanation of the study, which included information about radiation exposure during the CT examinations, was given to all patients. Exclusion criteria were respiratory dysfunction and previous reactions to iodinated contrast media. Fifty-six consecutive patients (31 men and 25 women; mean age, 51 years; range, 37–66 years) all with solitary pulmonary nodules were enrolled prospectively in the study. Pathological diagnoses were acquired by CT-guided puncture biopsy or surgical resection or bronchofibroscopic biopsy within 2 weeks before or after the CT perfusion was performed (32 malignant: 11 squamous cell carcinoma, 6 adeno-squamous carcinoma, 11 adeno carcinoma, and 4 small cell lung carcinoma; 24 benign: 7 inflammatory pseudotumour, 8 tuberculoma, 4 hamartoma, 4 global atelectasis, 1 sclerosing angioma). Mean tumour size was 10.7 cm³, ranging from 2.4 cm³ to 44.1 cm³.

The radiation dose of the dynamic CT was calculated from the dose–length product (DLP) listed in the exposure summary sheet generated by the CT equipment and multiplied by a k-factor of 0.014 [8].

CT perfusion imaging technique

Before the examination, all patients underwent breath exercise training to ensure that they could hold their breath for the duration of the entire perfusion procedure (approximately 30 s). Shallow abdominal breathing was permitted at the end stage of acquisition in cases where the patients were unable to hold their breath for the entire period of CT data acquisition. Two 20-gauge intravenous catheters were placed, one in each antecubital vein.

Before perfusion CT, unenhanced helical CT of the entire thorax was performed to determine the location of the SPN. The dynamic volume CT perfusion was performed using 320-row multidetector CT (Aquilion ONE, Toshiba Medical Systems, Otawara, Japan) with z-axis coverage of 16 cm. With a dual-head power injector, 60 ml of non-ionic contrast medium with an iodine concentration of 370 mg I/ml (Iopromide, Bayer Schering, Berlin, Germany) was injected at a flow rate of 8 ml/s (4 ml/s on each side). Two seconds after the start of the bolus injection, 15 intermittent low-dose volume acquisitions were made with 2-s intervals with no table movement.

The dynamic volume CT protocol was performed with the following parameters: 80-kV tube voltage, 80-mA tube current, 0.5-s gantry rotation speed, and 0.5-mm slice thickness. The 16-cm coverage included both the lung hilum and the SPN. The first two volumes were acquired before the contrast medium arrived in the heart and served as a baseline. The duration of the breath hold was approximately 30 s. The data were processed with adaptive iterative dose reduction (AIDR 3D) and automatically reconstructed with 0.5-mm slice thickness and 0.5-mm spacing, resulting in 320 images per volume and a total of 4,800 images for the entire perfusion data set.

Data post-processing and analysis

Post-processing was performed using perfusion software available on the CT equipment (Body Perfusion, dual-

Eur Radiol (2013) 23:2469–2474

input maximum slope analysis, Toshiba Medical Systems, Otawara, Japan). The first step is volume registration. The registration is performed to correct for motion between the dynamic volumes and creates a registered volume series. The registered volumes were then loaded into the body perfusion analysis software.

Rectangular ROIs (mean area 1.0 cm^2) were manually placed in the pulmonary artery trunk and the aorta at the level of the hilum to generate the TDCs representing the PA input function and the BA input function respectively. An elliptical ROI was placed in the left atrium, and the peak time of the left atrium TDC was used to differentiate pulmonary circulation (before the peak time point) and bronchial circulation (after the peak time point) [2]. A freehand ROI was drawn to encompass the lesion to generate the TDC of the contrast medium's first-pass attenuation in the SPN. The perfusion analysis range was set from 0 HU to 150 HU to restrict the perfusion analysis to soft tissue regions only and to ignore lung parenchyma and bone. Finally, 512×512 matrix colour-coded maps of the PF, BF and PI (PI = PF/(PF + BF)) were generated automatically. For each lesion, measurements were repeated on all relevant 5.0-mm axial slices and then averaged to calculate the final value. Tumour volume (size) was measured on commercial software (organ selection, Vitrea version 6.0, Vital Images, Minnetonka, MN, USA).

Statistical analysis

Statistical analysis was performed using commercially available software (SPSS, V13.0). Student's t test and the 95 % confidence interval were used to compare perfusion parameters between malignant and benign. ROC analysis was used to calculate and compare the diagnostic values of the three perfusion parameters in identifying lung cancer. A P value lower than 0.05 was considered to indicate a significant difference.

Results

Eleven patients adopted shallow abdominal breathing because of hypoxia at the end stage of the perfusion CT. All patients showed good compliance with the CT perfusion procedure despite the relatively high injection rate of contrast agent and the slightly long breath-hold duration of 30 s. No severe adverse events occurred.

Perfusion parameters were visualised by colour maps and fused onto the original axial CT images. Representative perfusion colour maps are shown in Figs. 1 and 2. Perfusion results of the 56 SPNs derived from DI-CTP are listed in Table 1 and shown in Fig. 3. Of the 56 SPNs, significant differences in all three perfusion parameters were revealed between malignant and benign tumours. The PI demonstrates the greatest difference between malignant and benign: 0.30± 0.07 vs. 0.51±0.13 , $P<0.001$. The area under the ROC of the PI is 0.92, the largest of the three perfusion parameters, indicating a sensitivity of 0.95, specificity of 0.83, +LR of 5.59, and –LR of 0.06 for identifying lung cancer. The dynamic perfusion protocol was identical for all 56 cases. The CT dose DLP=324.8 mGy. cm or 4.55 mSv (k=0.014).

Discussion

In vivo measurement of the two circulations in lung cancer was not technically possible until recently. Bronchial blood flow in lung cancer has been confirmed by many reports from bronchoangiography studies [9]. On the other hand, in vivo evidence of pulmonary circulation in lung cancer was

Fig. 1 Axial coloured perfusion maps in a 48-year-old male patient with inflammatory pseudotumour located in the left inferior lung (*arrowhead*). Nearly balanced perfusion between pulmonary circulation and bronchial circulation was demonstrated in this case

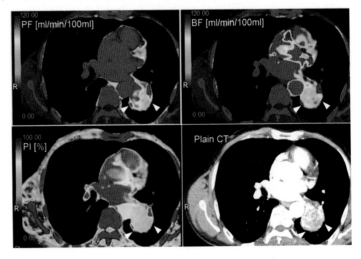

Fig. 2 Axial coloured perfusion maps in a 58-year-old male patient with adenocarcinoma located in the left superior lung. The perfusion is heterogeneous throughout the tumour. Bronchial circulation is globally dominant, especially in the gastro part of the tumour (*arrow*)

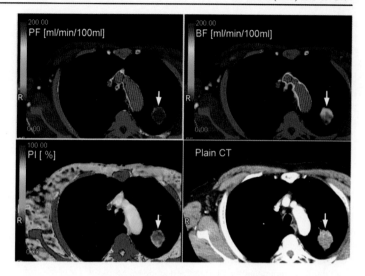

rarely documented, except for a hint from a previous study [10], which reported that some lung cancer tumours enhanced earlier than the enhancement of the aorta, indicating significant blood flow from pulmonary vessels. Theoretically, the single-input maximum slope algorithm calculates blood flow as the ratio of (maximum slope of the tissue TDC)/(maximum HU of the feeding artery). In the case of a double vascular system, such as pulmonary and bronchial circulation in lung tumours, the maximum slope in the tissue's TDC represents the dominant blood flow; the lower blood flow is thus ignored by single-input analysis. Considering that bronchial or systemic blood flow is relatively higher than the pulmonary blood flow in lung cancer (Figs. 2 and 3), the single-input maximum slope analysis result is just the bronchial flow. Vice versa, the blood flow in benign tumours derived from the single-input maximum slope analysis is the pulmonary blood flow. Insufficient assessment of the lung tumour's true haemodynamics may be the reason why the diagnostic performance of CT perfusion in lung cancer reported previously [11] is not as good as the figures

from this study. In this study, in all cases the blood flow fractions of the two circulations are heterogeneous within the tumour (Fig. 2); regional measurement therefore differs significantly from whole volume assessment. This may be another reason for the difference in the findings between this investigation and previously reported studies, which were performed within one or two transverse CT sections owing to the limited detector width of the device.

In terms of the total blood flow in normal lung tissue, the bronchial blood flow fraction is very low, to the order of 1 % to 2 %. However, the bronchial blood flow is crucial for maintaining airway and lung function [12] and is more transformable under pathological conditions. In lung cancer the BA fraction increases. Findings from this study support a dominant bronchial blood flow with a relatively low fraction of pulmonary blood flow in malignant SPNs (Table 1, Figs. 2 and 3), as demonstrated by the PI=0.30±0.07 derived from DI-CTP. For benign tumours, nearly balanced perfusion between pulmonary circulation and bronchial circulation was demonstrated with a PI of 0.51±0.13. These findings may

Table 1 Perfusion and receiver-operating characteristic (ROC) analysis results

Perfusion parameters		n	Mean	SD	95 % CI		t test	Area under ROC (95 % CI)
					Lower	Upper		
PF (ml/min/100 ml)	Malignant	32	24.56	10.85	20.65	28.47	$P<0.001$	0.85
	Benign	24	44.88	16.01	38.12	51.64		(0.75–0.96)
BF (ml/min/100 ml)	Malignant	32	58.17	26.78	48.51	67.82	$P=0.028$	0.66
	Benign	24	43.32	20.56	34.64	52.00		(0.52–0.81)
PI (100 %)	Malignant	32	0.30	0.07	0.27	0.33	$P<0.001$	0.92
	Benign	24	0.51	0.13	0.46	0.57		(0.85–1.00)

PF pulmonary flow, *BF* bronchial flow, *PI* perfusion index

Springer

Eur Radiol (2013) 23:2469–2474

not only benefit the differential diagnosis of lung cancer, but also help lung cancer treatment planning: (1) If interventional therapy is a choice for patients with lung cancer, we can make the decision whether transpulmonary artery treatment or transbronchial artery treatment will be performed based on the value of the PI. (2) Because of different oxygen concentrations in pulmonary and systemic blood, the PI does indicate oxygen saturation in the tumour by considering the BA fraction. It has been reported that a high level of oxygenation leads to greater radiosensitivity [13]. The PI is potentially useful for forecasting the therapeutic effect of radiotherapy treatment in lung cancers.

Receiver-operating characteristic curve analysis is used to assess the diagnostic performance of a certain index for a certain disease state, the area under the curve indicating its diagnostic efficiency: the larger the area, the better the diagnostic performance [14]. Among the ROC curves of the three perfusion parameters, the PI has the largest area under its curve, indicating the PI as the best among the three for discriminating between malignant and benign (Fig. 4). To further determine its sensitivity and specificity, a cutoff value point in the curve was determined. Usually this point is defined as having the shortest distance to the left upper corner of the ROC coordinate system. In this study the cutoff value of PI is 0.42, generating sensitivity of 0.95, specificity of 0.83, +LR of 5.59, and –LR of 0.06. The positive and negative predictive values (PPVs and NPVs) of a test in confirming and excluding a diagnosis of cancer in a group of patients depend on the prevalence of cancer in that group. In contrast, the –LR and +LR were regarded as

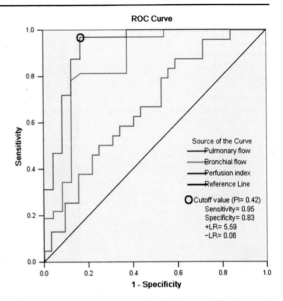

Fig. 4 Receiver-operating characteristic (ROC) curves of the three perfusion parameters for identifying lung cancer. The cutoff value of the perfusion index (PI) is defined as the point with the shortest distance to the left upper corner of the ROC coordinate system (toroid). $-LR = (1 - \text{sensitivity})/\text{specificity}$ and $+LR = \text{sensitivity}/(1 - \text{specificity})$

being more stable than PPVs and NPVs in delineating diagnostic efficiency and therefore were chosen in this study [15, 16]. When the +LR has a value >10 and –LR<0.1, we have great confidence in confirming or ruling out a certain disease. Accordingly, if a case of SPN has a PI value higher than 0.42 the cancer diagnosis can be ruled out with great confidence.

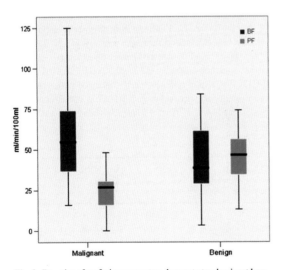

Fig. 3 Box plot of perfusion parameters demonstrates dominant bronchial circulation along with relatively low pulmonary circulation in lung cancers and nearly balanced perfusion between the two circulations in benign lung tumours

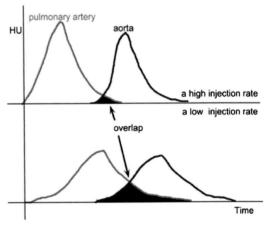

Fig. 5 For a fixed total contrast agent volume, a higher injection rate means shorter injection duration resulting in sharper shapes of the TDCs of the two input arteries, therefore leading to less overlap in the phase domain between these two circulations

 Springer

2474

Eur Radiol (2013) 23:2469–2474

However if the PI value is lower than 0.42, the lung cancer diagnosis can be suggested, but without too much confidence owing to a relatively low +LR. Further tests, such as biopsy, should be adopted to confirm the diagnosis.

There are limitations to this study. The overlap of the two circulations may undermine the validity of the perfusion measurements. A high injection rate and therefore short injection duration was achieved to reduce such overlap by bolus injection of CM through the left and right antecubital veins (Fig. 5) [2]. The integration of the diagnostic information from CT morphology and perfusion was proposed to be more helpful in the differential diagnosis than using perfusion measurements alone [17]. Thus, the usefulness of the integration of CT morphology and DI-CTP needs to be assessed further. Considering the diversity of the pathological types of lung tumours and differences in haemodynamics in various pathological conditions, the relatively small sample size of this investigation will unavoidably lead to selection bias and therefore biased results to some extent. Therefore, population-based investigation is warranted to further determine the clinical utility of these findings. The radiation exposure is an inherent limitation of perfusion CT, which increases with tube voltage, tube current, and the number of CT volume exposures. In order to keep the overall radiation dose within the range of clinical utility, we reduced the kV and mA in CT perfusion so that the dose was comparable with a triphasic abdominal imaging procedure [18, 19].

In conclusion, the PI derived from dual-input maximum slope CT perfusion, which represents the fraction of pulmonary circulation and systemic circulation in SPNs, is a useful biomarker for identifying malignancy vs. benignity in solitary pulmonary nodules. The perfusion index may be potentially useful for lung cancer treatment planning and forecasting the therapeutic effect of radiotherapy treatment.

Acknowledgements The authors thank Dr. Kolo of Toshiba Medical Systems for outstanding technical assistance in this study.

Xiadong Yuan and Jing Zhang contributed equally to this work.

References

1. Milne EN (1967) Circulation of primary and metastatic pulmonary neoplasms: a postmortem microarteriographic study. Am J Roentgenol Radium Ther Nucl Med 100:603–619

2. Yuan X, Zhang J, Ao G et al (2012) Lung cancer perfusion: can we measure pulmonary and bronchial circulation simultaneously? Eur Radiol 22:1665–1671

3. Nair A, Hansell DM (2011) European and North American lung cancer screening experience and implications for pulmonary nodule management. Eur Radiol 21:2445–2454

4. Sitartchouk I, Roberts HC, Pereira AM et al (2008) Computed tomography perfusion using first pass methods for lung nodule characterization. Invest Radiol 43:349–358

5. Li Y, Yang ZG, Chen TW et al (2010) First-pass perfusion imaging of solitary pulmonary nodules with 64-detector row CT: comparison of perfusion parameters of malignant and benign lesions. Br J Radiol 83:785–790

6. Zhang M, Kono M (1997) Solitary pulmonary nodules: evaluation of blood flow patterns with dynamic CT. Radiology 205:471–478

7. Lee YH, Kwon W, Kim MS et al (2010) Lung perfusion CT: the differentiation of cavitary mass. Eur J Radiol 73:59–65

8. Valentin J (2007) Managing patient dose in multi-detector computed tomography (MDCT). Ann ICRP 37:1–79

9. Luo L, Wang H, Ma H et al (2010) Analysis of 41 cases of primary hypervascular non-small cell lung cancer treated with embolization of emulsion of chemotherapeutics and iodized oil. Zhongguo Fei Ai Za Zhi 13:540–543

10. Kiessling F, Boese J, Corvinus C (2004) Perfusion CT in patients with advanced bronchial carcinomas: a novel chance for characterization and treatment monitoring? Eur Radiol 14:1226–1233

11. Ohno Y, Koyama H, Matsumoto K et al (2011) Differentiation of malignant and benign pulmonary nodules with quantitative first-pass 320-detector row perfusion CT versus FDG PET/CT. Radiology 258:599–609

12. McCullagh A, Rosenthal M, Wanner A et al (2010) The bronchial circulation–worth a closer look: a review of the relationship between the bronchial vasculature and airway inflammation. Pediatr Pulmonol 45:1–13

13. Wang J, Ning W, Cham MD et al (2009) Tumor response in patients with advanced non–small cell lung cancer: perfusion CT evaluation of chemotherapy and radiation therapy. AJR Am J Roentgenol 193:1090–1096

14. He H, Lyness JM, McDermott MP (2009) Direct estimation of the area under the receiver operating characteristic curve in the presence of verification bias. Stat Med 28:361–376

15. Goehring C, Perrier A, Morabia A (2004) Spectrum bias: a quantitative and graphical analysis of the variability of medical diagnostic test performance. Stat Med 23:125–135

16. Bhandari M, Guyatt GH (2005) How to appraise a diagnostic test. World J Surg 29:561–566

17. Marten K, Grabbe E (2003) The challenge of the solitary pulmonary nodule: diagnostic assessment with multislice spiral CT. Clin Imaging 27:156–161

18. Tsai HY, Tung CJ, Yu CC, Tyan YS (2007) Survey of computed tomography scanners in Taiwan: dose descriptors, dose guidance levels, and effective doses. Med Phys 34:1234–1243

19. Galanski M, Nagel HD, Stamm G (2007) Results of a federation inquiry 2005/2006: pediatric CT X-ray practice in Germany. Rofo 179:1110–1111

ORIGINAL RESEARCH ■ **TECHNICAL DEVELOPMENTS**

Radiology

A Simplified Whole-Organ CT Perfusion Technique with Biphasic Acquisition: Preliminary Investigation of Accuracy and Protocol Feasibility in Kidneys[1]

XiaoDong Yuan, MD, PhD
Jing Zhang, MD, PhD
ChangBin Quan, MD
Yuan Tian, MD
Hong Li, MD
GuoKun Ao, MD

Purpose: To determine the feasibility and accuracy of a protocol for calculating whole-organ renal perfusion (renal blood flow [RBF]) and regional perfusion on the basis of biphasic computed tomography (CT), with concurrent dynamic contrast material–enhanced (DCE) CT perfusion serving as the reference standard.

Materials and Methods: This prospective study was approved by the institutional review board, and written informed consent was obtained from all patients. Biphasic CT of the kidneys, including precontrast and arterial phase imaging, was integrated with a first-pass dynamic volume CT protocol and performed and analyzed in 23 patients suspected of having renal artery stenosis. The perfusion value derived from biphasic CT was calculated as CT number enhancement divided by the area under the arterial input function and compared with the DCE CT perfusion data by using the paired *t* test, correlation analysis, and Bland-Altman plots. Correlation analysis was made between the RBF and the extent of renal artery stenosis. All postprocessing was independently performed by two observers and then averaged as the final result.

Results: Mean ± standard deviation biphasic and DCE CT perfusion data for RBF were 425.62 mL/min ± 124.74 and 419.81 mL/min ± 121.13, respectively ($P = .53$), and for regional perfusion they were 271.15 mL/min per 100 mL ± 82.21 and 266.33 mL/min per 100 mL ± 74.40, respectively ($P = .31$). Good correlation and agreement were shown between biphasic and DCE CT perfusion for RBF ($r = 0.93$; ±10% variation from mean perfusion data [$P < .001$]) and for regional perfusion ($r = 0.90$; ±13% variation from mean perfusion data [$P < .001$]). The extent of renal artery stenosis was negatively correlated with RBF with biphasic CT perfusion ($r = -0.81$, $P = .012$).

Conclusion: Biphasic CT perfusion is clinically feasible and provides perfusion data comparable to DCE CT perfusion data at both global and regional levels in the kidney.

Online supplemental material is available for this article.

[1] From the Department of Radiology, the 309th Hospital of Chinese People's Liberation Army, 17 Heishanhu Rd, Haidian District, Beijing 100091, P.R. China. Received November 30, 2014; revision requested January 5, 2015; revision received May 8; accepted June 12; final version accepted July 21. Supported by the Beijing Municipal Science and Technology Commission (grant Z131107002213076) and our institution (grant 2013ZD-005). **Address correspondence to** G.A. (e-mail: *aoguokun309@163.com*).

Radiology

Dynamic contrast material–enhanced (DCE) wide-coverage computed tomography (CT), such as the "shuttle-scan" and the dynamic wide-area detector volume CT techniques (1–3), expands traditional regional CT perfusion to whole-organ CT perfusion, thereby providing comprehensive perfusion information. However, whole-organ perfusion at CT exposes a large volume of tissue to additional radiation exposure, resulting in a higher radiation dose and longer acquisition time (4). CT perfusion requires dynamic CT acquisition, typically 10–20 intermittent scans with 1–2-second intervals during a breath hold of 20–30 seconds. It is difficult to integrate such dynamic scanning of a whole organ into a routine multiphasic CT examination. These factors, have, perhaps, contributed to the slow adoption of whole-organ CT perfusion techniques.

By employing the Fick principle (5,6) in a single-compartment model with no venous outflow, one can extract perfusion data (blood flow) by dividing the increase in CT numbers by the area under the arterial input function (AIF). Thus, we hypothesized that renal perfusion (or renal blood flow [RBF]) and regional perfusion data can be obtained by using biphasic CT with single-section tracking images. We designed this investigation to determine the protocol feasibility and accuracy of a biphasic CT perfusion technique in the kidney, with DCE CT perfusion serving as the reference standard.

Materials and Methods

Subjects

This prospective study was approved by our institutional review board, and written informed consent was obtained from all patients. Between January and October 2014, 25 consecutive patients (mean age ± standard deviation, 54.1 years ± 10.7; range, 32–77 years) suspected of having renal artery stenosis (RAS) were enrolled, among whom 14 patients had unexplained, severe, or rapidly progressive hypertension, and 11 patients were suspected of having RAS on the basis of ultrasonographic (US) imaging. Fourteen patients were men (mean age, 53.6 years ± 12.5; range, 32–75 years), and 11 were women (mean age, 54.7 years ± 9.4; range, 35–77 years). Patients were selected for this study in accordance with the following criteria: *(a)* suspicion of RAS and referral for biphasic CT evaluation by clinicians, *(b)* no contraindications to the administration of iodinated contrast media. Two men (70 and 68 years old) were excluded from data analyses after CT imaging, one because of severe motion artifacts, and the other because of incomplete imaging of the kidneys due to a z-axis dimension greater than the limit of the 16-cm coverage of the 320–detector row CT scanner. The remaining 23 patients, (12 men and 11 women, 46 kidneys) were included in the perfusion analysis and statistical comparison of biphasic and DCE CT perfusion.

Combined Protocol of Biphasic CT and First-Pass Dynamic Volume CT

Biphasic CT was incorporated in a modified DCE CT perfusion protocol (7) in which tube-current–boosted arterial-phase imaging was performed as part of the dynamic volume CT protocol and triggered with a fixed delay time after the initial enhancement of the abdominal aorta (Fig 1). A 320–detector row CT scanner (Aquilion ONE; Toshiba Medical Systems Corporation, Otawara, Japan) was used. First, precontrast helical CT of the abdomen with breath hold was performed from the top of the left diaphragm to the pelvic inlet at end inspiration with tube-current modulation at 100 kV. Then, a power injector was used for administration of 44 mL (for patients < 70 kg of body weight) or 55 mL (for patients with ≥ 70 kg of body weight) of iodinated contrast material (Iopromide, 370 mg of iodine per milliliter; Bayer Schering, Berlin, Germany). The injection was given via a cubital vein at a rate of 4.0 mL/sec and 5.0 mL/sec, respectively, for patients in

Advances in Knowledge

■ The biphasic CT perfusion technique is clinically and technically feasible and provides perfusion data comparable to that of dynamic contrast–enhanced CT perfusion at both global and regional levels in the kidney (renal blood flow, $r = 0.93$; $[P < .001]$; renal perfusion, $r = 0.90$; $[P < .001]$).

■ Renal blood flow derived from biphasic CT perfusion data demonstrated good correlation ($r = -0.81$, $P = .012$) with the severity of renal artery stenosis ($r = -0.81$, $P = .012$).

Implications for Patient Care

■ The presented biphasic CT perfusion technique can allow reduction of patient radiation dose by 75%, because it involves only one contrast-enhanced scan instead of the repeated scans required with the dynamic contrast-enhanced CT.

■ A lengthy breath hold is not necessary for the proposed technique, resulting in good patient compliance and a reduction in motion artifacts compared with those with dynamic contrast-enhanced CT perfusion.

Published online before print
10.1148/radiol.2015142757   Content code: CT

Radiology 2016; 279:254–261

Abbreviations:
AIF = arterial input function
DCE = dynamic contrast material enhanced
RAS = renal artery stenosis
RBF = renal blood flow

Author contributions:
Guarantor of integrity of entire study, X.Y.; study concepts/study design or data acquisition or data analysis/interpretation, all authors; manuscript drafting or manuscript revision for important intellectual content, all authors; approval of final version of submitted manuscript, all authors; agrees to ensure any questions related to the work are appropriately resolved, all authors; literature research, X.Y., Y.T., H.L., G.A.; clinical studies, X.Y., J.Z., H.L., G.A.; experimental studies, X.Y., J.Z., C.Q., G.A.; statistical analysis, J.Z., C.Q., Y.T.; and manuscript editing, C.Q., Y.T., H.L., G.A.

Conflicts of interest are listed at the end of this article.

Radiology

Figure 1

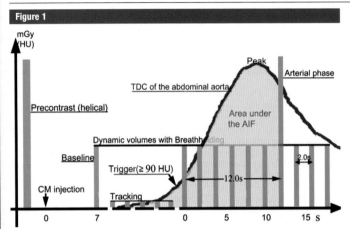

Figure 1: Graph shows time sequence display of combined protocol for biphasic CT and dynamic volume CT. Shadow area represents area under the AIF. Dynamic volume imaging included one baseline volume scan and 10 intermittent volumetric cine scans. Seventh scan (arterial phase) was performed 12 seconds after beginning of cine scan (ie, 12 seconds after initial enhancement [≥ 90 HU] of abdominal aorta). Because contrast material injection duration was fixed at 11 seconds, arterial phase acquisition was most likely to occur at peak time point of abdominal aorta or slightly later (2–3 seconds). CM = contrast material, TDC = time-density curve.

the two weight groups, with a fixed injection duration of 11 seconds, followed by 20 mL of saline solution at the same rate. At 7 seconds after the beginning of the injection, the first volume scan (baseline) of the dynamic series was performed at end inspiration, followed by a single-section tracking series (section thickness, 5 mm; tube current, 90 mA; voltage, 100 kV) at the renal hilum level. Then, the volumetric cine scans were automatically triggered at a preset threshold of greater than or equal to 90 HU in the lumen of the abdominal aorta. Ten intermittent breath-hold volumetric cine scans every 2 seconds were then performed without table movement. The seventh volume scan, 12 seconds after the beginning of the volumetric cine series, was performed at 300 mA to produce the arterial phase images for diagnosis and analysis of biphasic CT. The dynamic volumetric cine series and the baseline volume scan were used to calculate DCE CT perfusion. The scan range was fixed at 16 cm to include both kidneys in this range along the z-axis. The scan parameters

were collimation, 320 × 0.5 mm; voltage, 100 kV; tube current, 90 mA (300 mA for the seventh volume series); gantry rotation time, 0.35 seconds; matrix, 512 × 512; and field of view, 300–350 mm. All patients were asked to hold their breath before the baseline volume scan. The duration of the breath hold was from the baseline volume scan through the tracking process to the end of the dynamic volumetric cine scans, approximately 24 seconds. The data were processed with adaptive iterative dose reduction and were reconstructed automatically with a section thickness of 5 mm and 5-mm spacing.

The volume CT dose index of the 11 dynamic volume scans displayed in the system dose summary was identical, at 28.0 mGy, for each patient. The anterior-posterior and lateral dimensions of the abdomen were measured on the anterior-posterior and lateral CT scanograms, respectively. The size-specific dose estimate conversion factors were determined by using the sum of both dimensions with a 32-cm diameter reference phantom (8). The

mean size-specific dose estimates of the dynamic volume CT were 38.53 mGy ± 8.56. The size-specific dose estimates of the arterial phase scan were 9.63 mGy ± 2.14, approximately 25% of the total dynamic volume CT dose. The size-specific dose estimates of the precontrast helical CT were 6.88 mGy ± 1.05.

DCE CT Perfusion Analysis

The volume registration was automatically performed with the body registration software (Toshiba Medical Systems Corporation, Otawara, Japan) and included the baseline volume scan and the 10 intermittent dynamic volume scans (a total of 11 volume scans). This was done to correct for motion between data acquisitions and to create a registered volume series. A single-input maximum slope model was used (9). A rectangular region of interest (mean area, 1.0 cm^2) was manually placed in the abdominal aorta at the level of the renal hilum to generate the time-density curve of the input artery. The perfusion analysis range was set at 0–80 HU to restrict the perfusion analysis to soft-tissue regions only. Finally, 512 × 512 matrix color-coded perfusion maps were generated automatically. For the RBF evaluation, a freehand region of interest was drawn on the perfusion map to encompass the renal parenchyma (including the cortex and medulla but avoiding vessels and fat tissue in the renal sinus and hilum, Fig 2) to generate the perfusion index in milliliters per minute per 100 mL; then, the RBF in milliliters per minute was generated for the current section and was calculated as the perfusion index times the cross-sectional area (in square centimeters) of the freehand zone times the section thickness of 0.5 cm. Such measurements were repeated for all relevant 5.0-mm axial sections and then summed to achieve the DCE CT perfusion RBF. For each kidney, one section (5.0 mm) at the hilum level was selected, and the corresponding perfusion index of the renal parenchyma was documented to represent DCE CT regional perfusion.

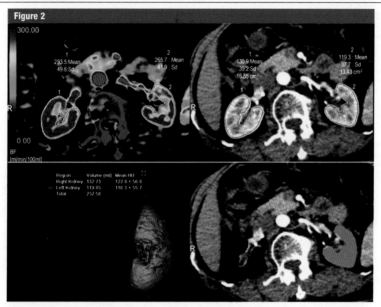

Figure 2: Perfusion maps derived from DCE CT perfusion imaging (upper images) show free-hand region of interest of renal parenchyma (including cortex and medulla) at the hilum level. Images generated during the biphasic CT perfusion analysis (lower images) show selection of whole kidney including cortex and medulla (lower right) as well as display of volume and average CT numbers of kidneys at arterial phase (lower left , shaded surface display) for calculating CT number increase used in biphasic CT perfusion calculation.

Biphasic CT Perfusion Analysis

According to the Fick principle,

$$Q = F \times \left[\int_0^t a(t) - \int_0^t v(t) \right],$$

where Q is the CT number increase, F is perfusion, $\int_0^t a(t)$ is the area under the arterial input function, and $\int_0^t v(t)$ is the area under the venous output function. With the hypothesis that there was no venous outflow, perfusion can be calculated as the maximum slope of tissue enhancement divided by the peak value of the input artery $[F = Q'/a(t)]$, namely the maximum slope method (10,11). By using the same principle and hypothesis, we proposed that with the biphasic CT perfusion technique,

perfusion can be determined as the CT number increase (Q) divided by the area under the arterial input function:

$$\left(F = \frac{Q}{\int_0^t a(t)} \right).$$

The arterial input function of renal perfusion was obtained from the images of the tracking process and the dynamic volume scans. Both the precontrast helical images and the arterial phase images were sent to a workstation (Vital Workstation, Vitrea version 6.0; Vital Images, Minnetonka, Minn), where the contours of the whole kidney (including the cortex and medulla) were automatically depicted with the organ selection tool and then manually edited in each section by using the edit tool to avoid including vessels and fat tissue in the renal sinus and hilum. Then the volume of each kidney

in milliliters (Vol_k) and corresponding mean CT numbers in Hounsfield units at both the precontrast and arterial phases were automatically determined (Fig 2). The product of the Vol_k and the CT number increase was calculated as: $Vol_k \times HU_{arterial} - Vol_k \times HU_{precontrast}$. The biphasic CT perfusion RBF was calculated as this product divided by the area (in Hounsfield units times minutes) under the AIF. For each kidney, one section from the arterial phase at the hilum level and the corresponding freehand region of interest (identical to those used in calculating the DCE CT regional perfusion) were chosen for calculating the biphasic CT regional perfusion. The CT number increase in this section was obtained by subtracting precontrast CT numbers in Hounsfield units from postcontrast CT numbers at the same z-axis level. The biphasic CT regional perfusion data were calculated as the CT number

Radiology

Perfusion Outcomes and Statistical Comparison between Biphasic CT Perfusion and DCE CT Perfusion

Perfusion Indexes	Perfusion Data	Difference	P Value	Pearson Correlation	P Value
RBF (mL/min)		5.81 ± 21.56 (−42.26, 42.26)*	.53	0.93	< .001
Biphasic CT	425.62 ± 124.74				
DCE CT	419.81 ± 121.13				
Regional perfusion (mL/min/100 mL)		4.82 ± 18.41 (−36.08, 36.08)†	.31	0.90	< .001
Biphasic CT	271.15 ± 82.21				
DCE CT	266.33 ± 74.40				

Note.—Unless otherwise indicated, data are means ± standard deviation, with 95% confidence intervals in parentheses (n = 46).

* Confidence intervals (Bland-Altman) are ± 10% of mean perfusion values.

† Confidence intervals (Bland-Altman) are ± 13% of mean perfusion values.

increase divided by the area (in Hounsfield units times minutes) under the AIF, and then multiplied by 100. The area under the AIF was estimated in spreadsheet software (Excel 2007; Microsoft, Redmond, Wash) by using the trapezoidal rule and the built-in sum and logical functions (if, and, or). The whole procedure described above, including the DCE CT perfusion and the biphasic CT perfusion analysis, was independently performed by two radiologists (X.Y. and J.Z, with 10 and 8 years of experience in CT perfusion, respectively) with each radiologist blinded to the results of the other. The final results were the average of those of both observers.

Assessment of Stenosis of the Renal Artery

The extent of RAS was quantitatively determined in the workstation from the arterial phase images. By using the vessel lumen assessment tools, the maximal stenosis site of the main renal artery and its corresponding minimum luminal diameter were automatically determined and manually corrected if necessary. The percentage of stenosis was calculated by the software as

$$(1 - \frac{S}{(R_1 + R_2)/2}) \times 100,$$

where S is the diameter of the stenosis, and R_1 and R_2 are the diameters of two reference sites manually set at portions of the main renal artery determined to

be normal that are proximal and distal to the lesion, respectively. This process was independently performed by the same two previously described readers (X.Y. and J.Z.), and their average provided the final value for analysis.

Statistical Analysis

The normal distribution test (Shapiro-Wilk test) was performed for four perfusion indexes (biphasic and DCE RBF, biphasic and DCE regional perfusion). The extent of the RAS percentage did not show a normal distribution. RBF and regional perfusion were compared between the biphasic and DCE CT perfusion scans by using the paired t test, Pearson correlation, and Bland-Altman plots. Spearman rank correlation was performed to compare biphasic CT perfusion RBF and the extent of RAS. If a kidney had an accessory renal artery, it was excluded from the correlation analysis between biphasic CT perfusion and the RAS. Interobserver reproducibility of biphasic CT RBF and biphasic CT regional perfusion was assessed by using Bland-Altman plots. Statistical analysis was performed by using commercially available software (SPSS 13.0; SPSS, Chicago, Ill). A P value of less than .05 was considered to indicate a significant difference.

Results

Of the 23 patients, 19 had RAS and 15 patients were affected bilaterally, among which three kidneys from three

patients were excluded from the correlation analysis between biphasic CT perfusion and RAS because of the presence of an accessory renal artery. On the basis of the arterial phase CT images in the 31 kidneys with arterial luminal stenosis (all caused by atherosclerosis) without an accessory renal artery, 21 were determined to have less than 50% stenosis, seven had 50%–70% stenosis, and three had more than 70% stenosis in diameter.

Perfusion results and the statistical comparison are displayed in the Table. Good correlation was demonstrated between the measurements of biphasic and DCE CT perfusion for RBF ($r = 0.93$, $P < .001$) (Fig 3a) and regional perfusion ($r = 0.90$, $P < .001$) (Fig 3b). The 95% confidence interval for the difference established with Bland-Altman plots showed a satisfying agreement between both techniques for RBF (95% confidence interval: −42.26, 42.26) and for regional perfusion (95% confidence interval: −36.08, 36.08) (Fig 4). Negative correlation was revealed by Spearman rank correlation analysis between biphasic CT RBF and the extent of RAS ($r = -0.81$, $P = .012$, Fig 5). The Bland-Altman plot analysis for interobserver agreement of biphasic CT RBF and regional perfusion and the percentage of stenosis of RAS showed that the 95% confidence intervals of the differences were −38.71, 38.71 mL/min; −32.45, 32.45 mL/min per 100 mL; and −9.12%, 9.12%, respectively (Figs E1–E3 [online]).

Radiology

Figure 3

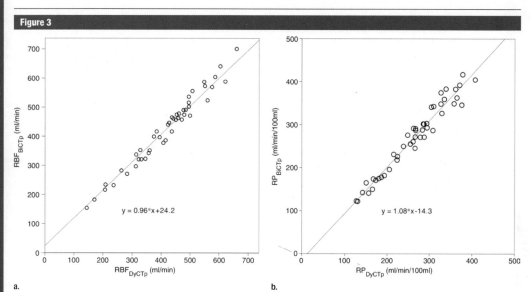

a.　　　　　　　　　　　　　　　　　　　　b.

Figure 3: Scatterplots show that correlation between biphasic CT perfusion (*BiCTp*) and DCE perfusion (*DyCTp*) for **(a)** RBF ($r = 0.93$, $P < .001$) and **(b)** regional perfusion (*RP*) ($r = 0.90$, $P < .001$) were high, with near-linear correlation ($y = 0.96 \cdot x + 24.2$ and $y = 1.08 \cdot x - 14.30$), respectively.

Figure 4

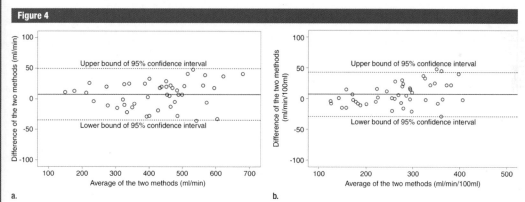

a.　　　　　　　　　　　　　　　　　　　　b.

Figure 4: Bland-Altman plots show that 95% confidence interval of the difference of the **(a)** RBF between the two methods was -42.26, 42.26 mL/min, which suggests that the maximum deviation of measurements between the two methods was approximately $\pm10\%$ of their averages and **(b)** regional perfusion between two methods was ±36.08 mL/min per 100 mL, which suggests that the maximum deviation of measurements between the two methods was approximately $\pm13\%$ of their averages.

Discussion

Similar to the maximum slope method, the biphasic CT perfusion technique uses the assumption of no venous outflow. Invalidation of this assumption results in an underestimation of perfusion. To meet this assumption, the CT perfusion technique must use a rapid injection rate and a relatively small volume of contrast material with a short injection duration. Usually, the injection duration should be less than 7 seconds, which may cause an increase in the incidence of contrast material extravasation and add to the cardiac burden of the examinees. Recently, results of a validation study (12) showed that the relatively

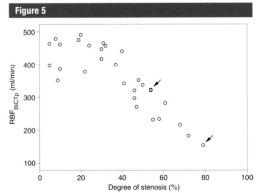

Figure 5

Figure 5: Scatterplot shows negative correlation between biphasic CT perfusion *(BiCTp)* RBF and extent of RAS (*n* = 31, *r* = −0.81, *P* = .012) as confirmed with Spearman rank correlation analysis. Nearly linear correlation was shown between them when the degree of stenosis was greater than 40% of diameter. Arrows denote two overlapping data points.

slow injection rate with 11.5 seconds used in a maximum slope perfusion CT protocol can lead to 8% underestimation of true perfusion. Therefore, DCE CT perfusion determined by using the maximum slope method that served as the reference standard in our study was likely to have caused slight underestimation of the true perfusion value because of the 11-second injection duration used in the protocol.

In the biphasic CT examination, the imaging during the arterial phase was performed (triggered) 12 seconds after the initial enhancement of the aorta (≥ 90 HU); this elapsed triggering time approximated the bolus injection duration of 11 seconds. According to the results of a previous study (13) and our experience, the time span from initial to peak enhancement of the aorta approximates the duration of contrast material injection. Therefore, the arterial phase acquisition was purposely designed to occur at the peak time point of the abdominal aorta or slightly later (2–3 seconds). There are two reasons for the timing of the arterial phase acquisition. First, according to our experience and those of authors of a previous study (14), the maximum enhancement of the renal cortex

usually occurs shortly after the peak enhancement of the aorta; therefore, such timing may allow a good signal-to-noise ratio. Second, later timing results in more venous outflow of the contrast material by the time of acquisition, leading to greater underestimation of perfusion.

The time-density curve of the abdominal aorta was used as the AIF in the analysis of biphasic CT perfusion. However the transmission delay of the bloodstream from the abdominal aorta to the renal parenchyma may have produced a time shift between the time-density curve of the abdominal aorta and the real AIF of renal perfusion, thus resulting in an underestimation of perfusion. In this investigation, both the RBF and the regional perfusion matched well between biphasic and DCE CT perfusion throughout a wide range of their values, which suggested that such a transmission delay for biphasic CT perfusion in assessment of renal perfusion was negligible. In addition, given that the accessory renal artery should have the same AIF as that for the abdominal aorta, the accuracy of biphasic CT perfusion should not be affected in patients with an accessory renal artery.

The degree of RAS typically correlates with RBF (15) and is often used to indicate the ischemic state of the kidney in clinical practice. Our results, as expected, mirrored the negative correlation between RBF and the extent of RAS; furthermore, we demonstrated no substantial decrease in RBF when the degree of stenosis was less than 40% and a linear decrease in RBF when the stenotic degree was greater than 40%.

The presented biphasic CT perfusion protocol has the following characteristics: *(a)* The tracking process starts a little earlier than usual and continues to obtain an AIF until the moment of the arterial phase acquisition. *(b)* A fast scan (volume or helical CT) should be initiated to capture the arterial phase of the kidneys in a short time, and no more than 1 second may be appropriate to minimize phase differences of the enhancement among different parts of the kidney. *(c)* No breath hold is required during the tracking process, because the abdominal aorta has no substantial movement with respiration. *(d)* Biphasic CT perfusion requires only one postcontrast acquisition; therefore, it can be performed with the same breath control strategy as that of the routine multiphasic CT and can allow substantial reduction in radiation dose to patients (75% radiation dose reduction in the present investigation compared with DCE CT perfusion).

Our study had a number of limitations. First, DCE CT perfusion with the maximum slope method is not a strong reference standard, although it has been validated in many previous studies (16,17). Second, the contrast material injection duration longer than that of a typical maximum slope CT perfusion protocol may have led to slight underestimation of perfusion. Third, the postcontrast scan required high temporal resolution for wide z-axis coverage to freeze the concentration of the iodinated contrast material in the target organ, so it may not be applicable to large organs. Fourth, a relatively small sample size with a high prevalence of RAS may have limited the ability to generalize from our results. Fifth, biphasic CT perfusion was only tested in the kidney and compared by using the maximum slope method. Tests in other organs or tumors with comparison to other perfusion analysis models may be necessary before generalization.

In conclusion, the biphasic CT perfusion protocol is clinically feasible and provides perfusion data comparable to that of DCE CT perfusion at both global and regional levels in the kidney.

Acknowledgments: The authors thank Kolo Pelesikoti, PhD, and Xu Yinghao, MS, of Toshiba Medical Systems for outstanding technical assistance in this study, and thank Weiwei Zhang, PhD, for language polishing.

Disclosures of Conflicts of Interest: X.Y disclosed no relevant relationships. **J.Z.** disclosed no relevant relationships. **C.Q.** disclosed no relevant relationships. **Y.T.** disclosed no relevant relationships. **H.L.** disclosed no relevant relationships. **G.A.** disclosed no relevant relationships.

References

1. Tacelli N, Remy-Jardin M, Copin MC, et al. Assessment of non-small cell lung cancer perfusion: pathologic-CT correlation in 15 patients. Radiology 2010;257(3):863–871.

2. Okada M, Kim T, Murakami T. Hepatocellular nodules in liver cirrhosis: state of the art CT evaluation (perfusion CT/volume helical shuttle scan/dual-energy CT, etc.). Abdom Imaging 2011;36(3):273–281.

3. Yuan X, Zhang J, Quan C, et al. Differentiation of malignant and benign pulmonary nodules with first-pass dual-input perfusion CT. Eur Radiol 2013;23(9):2469–2474.

4. Shankar JJ, Lum C, Sharma M. Whole-brain perfusion imaging with 320-MDCT scanner: Reducing radiation dose by increasing sampling interval. AJR Am J Roentgenol 2010; 195(5):1183–1186.

5. Peters AM, Gunasekera RD, Henderson BL, et al. Noninvasive measurement of blood flow and extraction fraction. Nucl Med Commun 1987;8(10):823–837.

6. Peters AM. Fundamentals of tracer kinetics for radiologists. Br J Radiol 1998;71(851): 1116–1129.

7. Kandel S, Kloeters C, Meyer H, Hein P, Hilbig A, Rogalla P. Whole-organ perfusion of the pancreas using dynamic volume CT in patients with primary pancreas carcinoma: acquisition technique, post-processing and initial results. Eur Radiol 2009;19(11):2641–2646.

8. Boone J, Strauss K, Cody D, et al. Size-specific dose estimates (SSDE) in pediatric and adult body CT examinations. Report of AAPM Task Group 204. College Park, Md: American Association of Physicists in Medicine, 2011.

9. Djuric-Stefanovic A, Saranovic Dj, Masulovic D, Ivanovic A, Pesko P. Comparison between the deconvolution and maximum slope 64-MDCT perfusion analysis of the esophageal cancer: is conversion possible? Eur J Radiol 2013;82(10):1716–1723.

10. Miles KA, Hayball MP, Dixon AK. Functional images of hepatic perfusion obtained with dynamic CT. Radiology 1993;188(2):405–411.

11. Miles KA, Griffiths MR. Perfusion CT: a worthwhile enhancement? Br J Radiol 2003; 76(904):220–231.

12. Kandel SM, Meyer H, Boehnert M, Hoppel B, Paul NS, Rogalla P. How influential is the duration of contrast material bolus injection in perfusion CT? evaluation in a swine model. Radiology 2014;270(1):125–130.

13. Bae KT. Peak contrast enhancement in CT and MR angiography: when does it occur and why? Pharmacokinetic study in a porcine model. Radiology 2003;227(3):809–816.

14. Helck A, Schönermarck U, Habicht A, et al. Determination of split renal function using dynamic CT-angiography: preliminary results. PLoS One 2014;9(3):e91774.

15. Zhang W, Qian Y, Lin J, Lv P, Karunanithi K, Zeng M. Hemodynamic analysis of renal artery stenosis using computational fluid dynamics technology based on unenhanced steady-state free precession magnetic resonance angiography: preliminary results. Int J Cardiovasc Imaging 2014;30(2):367–375.

16. Lemoine S, Papillard M, Belloi A, et al. Renal perfusion: noninvasive measurement with multidetector CT versus fluorescent microspheres in a pig model. Radiology 2011; 260(2):414–420.

17. Paul RK, Lum DP, Consigny DW, Grinde JR, Grist TM. CT perfusion in the treatment of a swine model of unilateral renal artery stenosis: validation with microspheres. J Vasc Interv Radiol 2009;20(4):513–523.